CW00646154

grooming

ESSENTIALS

for men

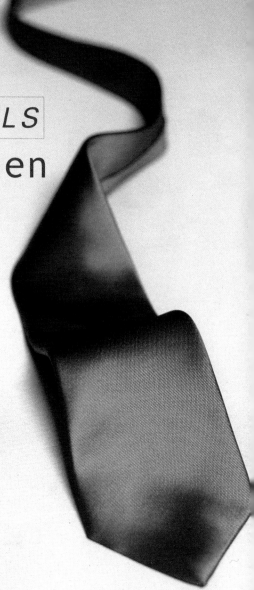

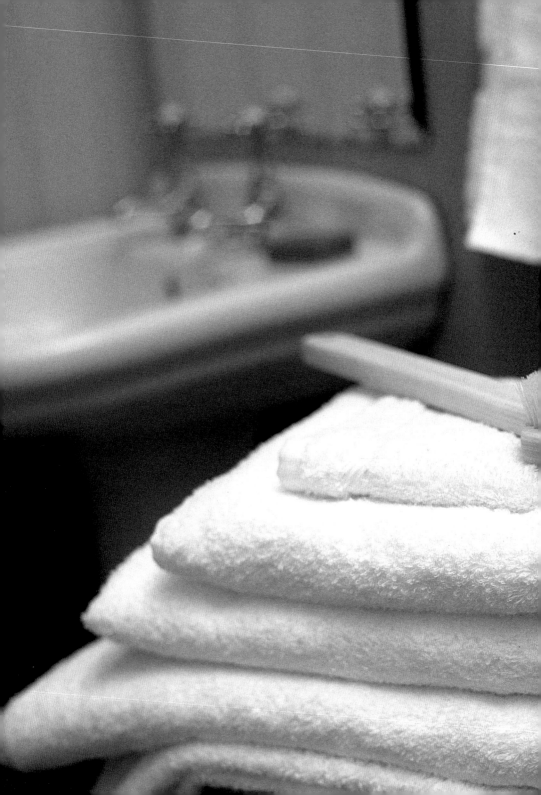

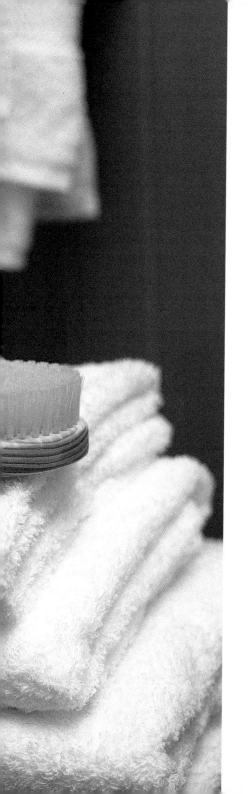

grooming

ESSENTIALS

for men

LOOKING GOOD AND FEELING GOOD

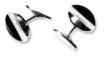

David Waters

CARLTON

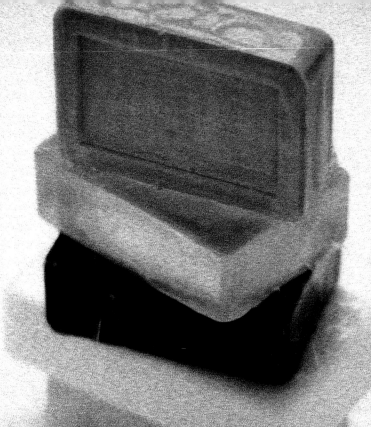

THIS IS A CARLTON BOOK

Text, design, special photography
and illustrations copyright © 1999
Carlton Books Limited

This edition published in 1999 by
Carlton Books Limited
20 St Anne's Court
Wardour Street
London W1V 3AW

A CIP catalogue for this book is available
from the British Library.

ISBN 1 85868 756 X

Printed and bound in Dubai.

Senior executive editor: Venetia Penfold
Art director: Penny Stock
Editor: Zia Mattocks
Senior art editor: Barbara Zuñiga
Designer: Liz Lewis
Picture researcher: Alex Pepper
Special photography: Jason Bell
Illustrations: Michael Hill
Production: Garry Lewis

contents

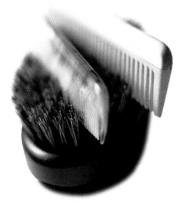

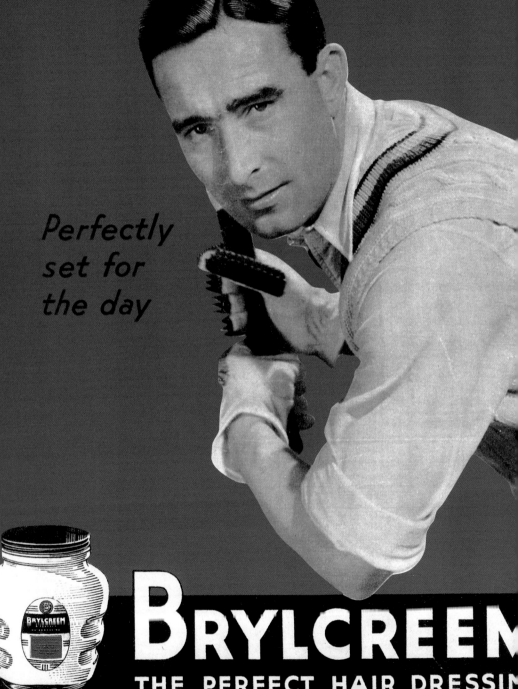

Perfectly
set for
the day

BRYLCREEM
THE PERFECT HAIR DRESSIN

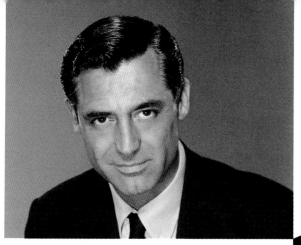

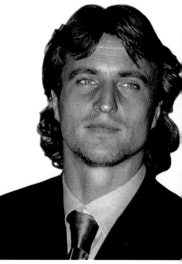

Introduction

In the late 1970s the boxer Henry Cooper encouraged us to buy a certain brand of aftershave by grunting, 'splash it all over'. So began and ended, pretty much, all men had to go on for grooming advice. It was not particularly useful information, especially when the product concerned smelt like something from a gym lost-property box, and applying it felt like you were sprinkling yourself with paint stripper. Men have been given very little advice since, hence the need for this long-overdue book.

Compare Henry's portrayal of spit-and-sawdust manhood with the kind of images that are used in men's fragrance advertising today. There is actor Rupert Everett pushing an upscale French fragrance reclining on a silk bed like an effete dandy. Or how about the row of androgynous youths and girls slouching around with tattoos and nose rings, challenging you to buy the latest unisex aroma from Calvin Klein? Even footballers, who have always had a macho image, have been transformed into style icons, and David Ginola is almost as famous for his mane of shiny hair as for his talent with the ball.

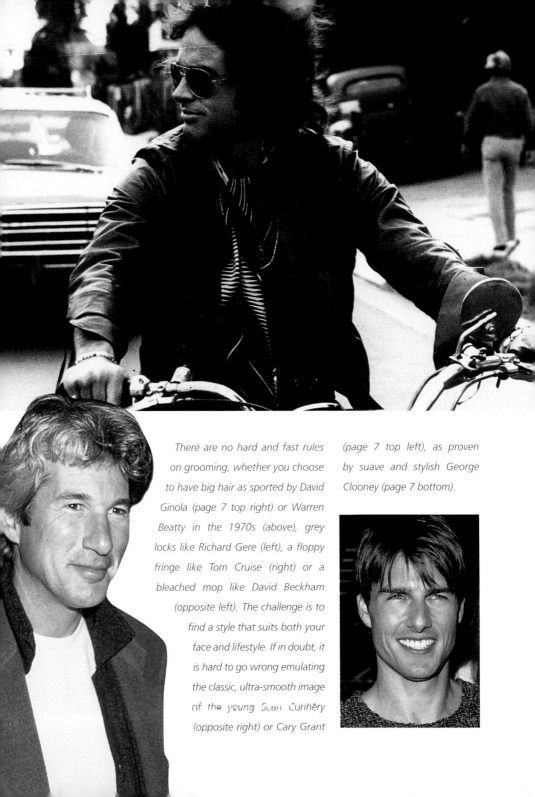

There are no hard and fast rules on grooming, whether you choose to have big hair as sported by David Ginola (page 7 top right) or Warren Beatty in the 1970s (above), grey locks like Richard Gere (left), a floppy fringe like Tom Cruise (right) or a bleached mop like David Beckham (opposite left). The challenge is to find a style that suits both your face and lifestyle. If in doubt, it is hard to go wrong emulating the classic, ultra-smooth image of the young Sean Connery (opposite right) or Cary Grant (page 7 top left), as proven by suave and stylish George Clooney (page 7 bottom).

Go to a grooming counter in any major department store or chemist and prepare to be amazed by the myriad of choices presented for men – from shaving balms and exfoliants to aromatherapy sports rubs and high sun-protection-factor skin creams. In the UK alone men are spending £800/$1,280 million a year on grooming products, but we have little notion of what we are buying, how to use these miracles in a bottle, and what they might actually do for us.

In researching this book I have drawn upon the latest information to bring together a detailed explanation of the world of grooming for men. We don't sit around like the women in our lives discussing the latest anti-wrinkle potions from Brand X, or debating good shaving techniques, sharing advice passed on from our fathers, and we certainly do not hand out the mini samples we have been given at the product counter. If we were happy doing that, there would be little need for this book. We get nervous discussing anything performed in the bathroom (apart from a particularly athletic tryst with a girlfriend involving a tub of ice cream). We find the subject of grooming unmanly and embarrassing, and although we still want to know what is out there and whether it will help us look a bit younger, or at least make our skin feel more comfortable, one thing is for sure: we are not going to get the information we need from our pals in a bar.

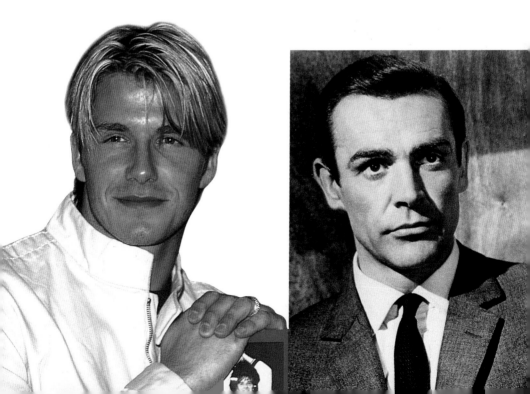

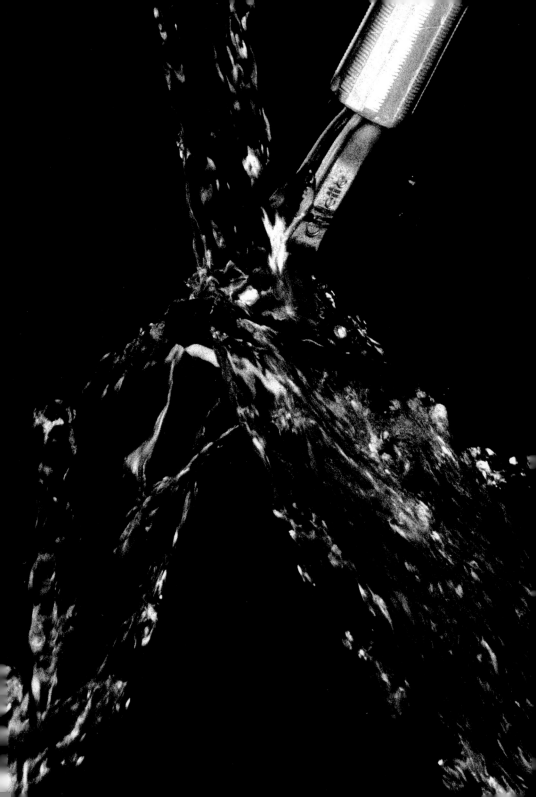

Chapter 1

the shave

NOTHING SYMBOLIZES BEING A MAN MORE THAN A DAILY SCRAPE AROUND THE CHIN WITH A SHARP IMPLEMENT. WOMEN DON'T DO IT, NEVER HAVE AND (HOPEFULLY) NEVER WILL. SHAVING IS ALSO A RITUAL AND NECESSITY THAT MANY OF US STILL HAVE NOT LEARNT TO DO WELL, WHICH IS WHY WE END UP LOOKING LIKE SHRAPNEL VICTIMS WITH SQUARES OF TISSUE DECORATING OUR CHINS ALMOST EVERY MORNING.

IN ADDITION TO REMOVING FACIAL HAIR, A DAILY SHAVE SHEARS OFF THE TOP LAYER OF DEAD SKIN CELLS, MAKING IT AN EFFECTIVE FORM OF EXFOLIATION. SHAVING REFRESHES YOUR SKIN, MAKES YOU LOOK WELL GROOMED AND IS OFTEN A MUST FOR WORK AND FOR CANOODLING WITH YOUR GIRLFRIEND. FURTHERMORE, ACCORDING TO ANTHROPOLOGISTS, A CLEAN-SHAVEN FACE IS A SIGN OF YOUTH AND VIRILITY.

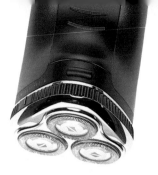

wet or dry?

SHAVING IS A BIT LIKE **WARFARE OR POLITICS** – men fall into one of two rival and mutually exclusive camps. Rare is the man who is happy to both wet and dry shave. On one side are the traditionalists, who promote the virtues of the old-fashioned wet shave and see their shaving results as highly superior to that of the modernists, who would prefer to stay in bed for an extra 15 minutes and love the latest electric gizmos that speed up their morning routines. If you can spare the time, join the ranks of the conservatives because a wet shave will always beat an electric one for smoothness and closeness – your face will feel fresher, too. The downside to wet shaving is the time it takes to do it properly. Yet for all its closeness, a wet shave cannot compete with the speed of an electric razor, which can remove the morning's stubble in a little over a minute – even while you are on the move (this is not a good idea, though). Recently, manufacturers of electric razors have significantly improved the closeness of the shave that can be achieved by their products, and some electric razors now even combine both wet and mechanical features.

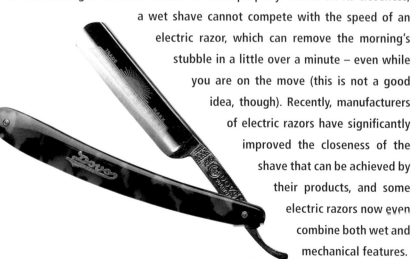

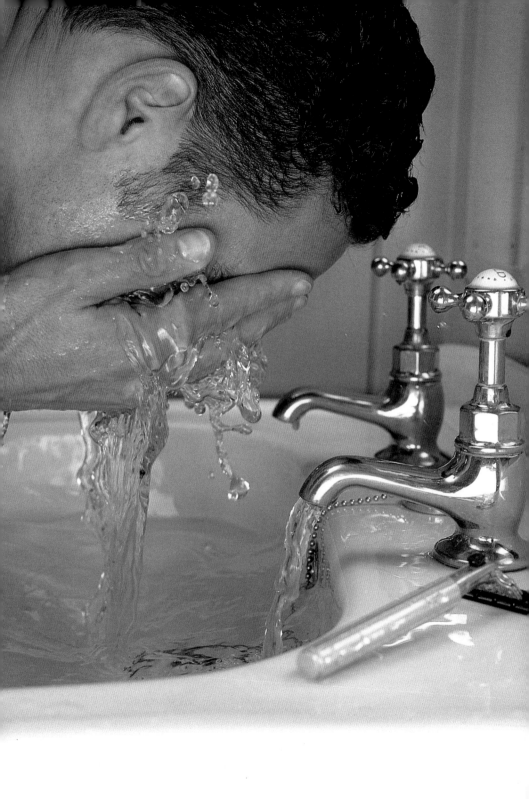

Slippery when wet

If you have strong, dark facial hair, the closer your morning shave, the smaller your chances will be of suffering from five-o'clock shadow (the annoying stubble that grows even before evening). If you need to look your best for a hot date, don't just shave twice in one day, it is too demanding on your skin and you will end up covered with unsightly nicks – the last thing you want when you are trying to make a good impression. Get up ten minutes earlier and get out your foam and blade. Following this guide to the best shaving equipment and techniques will help you achieve a smooth, close shave and make cutting yourself a thing of the past.

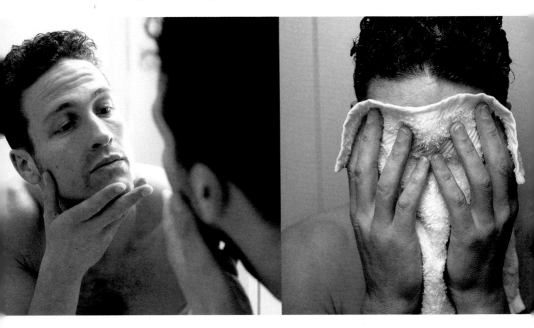

YOUR BEST-EVER SHAVE

Before you begin to do anything in the way of shaving, smooth your fingertips over your entire beard area to feel the direction of growth of your facial hair. You will find that mostly the beard grows downwards from your hairline towards your neck, but touch the area around your Adam's apple and feel how the hair there actually grows upwards. Whichever way your beard grows, the general rule is that this is the direction in which you should always shave.

Your allies in this battle against the unrelenting onslaught of facial hair are: hot water, a clean, sharp razor and plenty of lubrication – whether shaving foam, gel or oil. Start by splashing your face with several handfuls of almost-too-hot water; this softens the beard and the heat can actually expand the hair shaft by 30 per cent, making it easier for the blade to find. A face cloth soaked in extra-hot water, wrung out and placed over your neck and chin (where the growth is strongest) is also a good beard softener that makes shaving easier and more effective. Press the hot cloth into all the contours of your face, neck and chin, and leave it resting on your face for a few seconds to further expand the beard hairs.

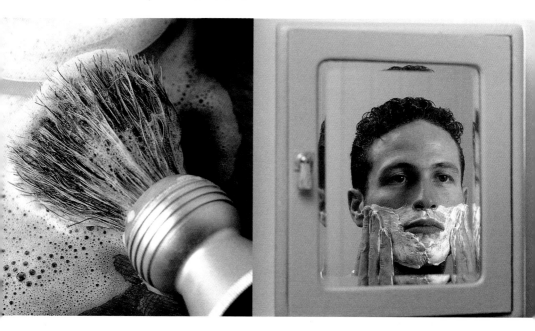

Gels are the most convenient moisteners, but foams and shaving soaps are good lubricators, too. Foams contain more air than gels and are therefore less protective against nicks and cuts than the denser gels. Applying your lubricant with a shaving brush, which you should rub vigorously over the beard area, helps lift the hairs away from the skin, making them easier to shave. If you have time to spare don't start shaving immediately, give the salve a couple of minutes to soften your beard first. Some men swear that applying moisturizer before the gel or foam softens the beard even more.

A swivel-headed razor with a two- or even a three-blade head will give you the closest shave. It should be replaced every three or four uses, depending on the thickness of your growth (heavier growth will wear out blades quicker). According to London hairdresser Daniel Rouah, using the same blade for a dozen shaves is equivalent to shaving with a shard of glass; give your skin a break and don't do it.

THE TECHNIQUE

Start shaving in slow but short downward sweeps with a steady pressure from the sides of your ears. The growth is less dense there and requires less lubrication, giving more time for your shaving foam to soften the tougher growth around your neck and chin. Then start shaving down your cheeks. Before reaching your chin, shave between your nose and top lip. The last areas you should shave are your chin and neck, which may require several sweeps of the razor to remove all the hair (check for stubble with your free hand). It will take some careful contortions of the blade to lift off all the hair and you may have to attack the beard in this particular spot with several different approaches, so forget the shaving-with-the-grain rule for the sake of a good result – but go carefully. Lastly, draw the razor under your jaw line and down your neck as far as your Adam's apple, using your free hand to check for any missed hairs. The final few strokes should be upwards from the beginning of your hair growth to the Adam's apple, since the hair is likely to grow towards your chin there.

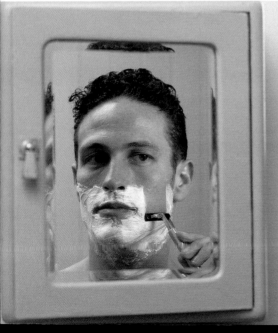
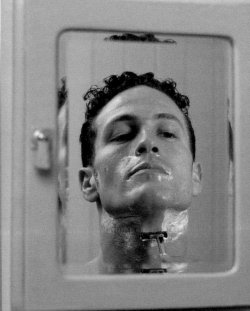

Throughout your shave use your free hand to gently pull and stretch your skin to create as-flat-as-possible surfaces for your razor blade. This will achieve a smoother shave and help avoid cutting your skin. Regularly rinse and tap the razor on the side of the sink or bath to remove the hair and foam build-up from the head. This will prevent the razor from clogging and keep the blade as sharp and clean as possible throughout.

Finally, smooth your hands all over your beard area to check for stray hairs and carefully reshave any places that you missed. When you have finished, rinse off the foam and splash your face several times with cold water to further rinse and refresh your skin.

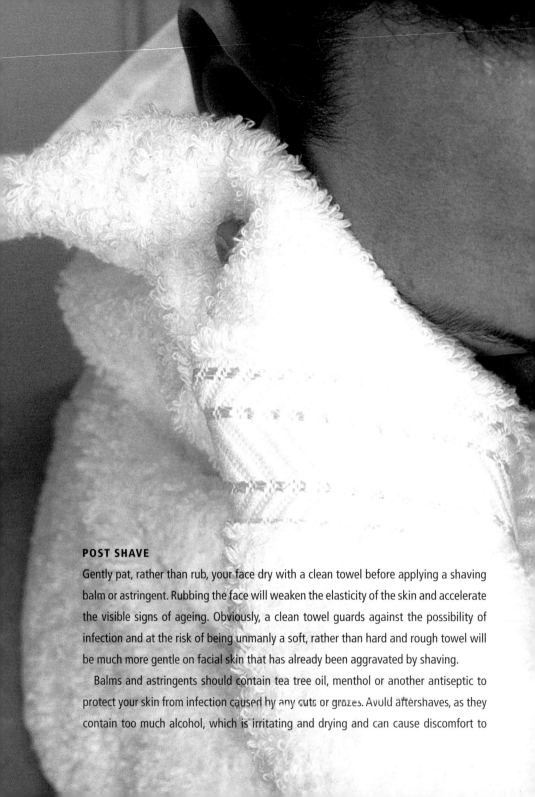

POST SHAVE

Gently pat, rather than rub, your face dry with a clean towel before applying a shaving balm or astringent. Rubbing the face will weaken the elasticity of the skin and accelerate the visible signs of ageing. Obviously, a clean towel guards against the possibility of infection and at the risk of being unmanly a soft, rather than hard and rough towel will be much more gentle on facial skin that has already been aggravated by shaving.

Balms and astringents should contain tea tree oil, menthol or another antiseptic to protect your skin from infection caused by any cuts or grazes. Avoid aftershaves, as they contain too much alcohol, which is irritating and drying and can cause discomfort to

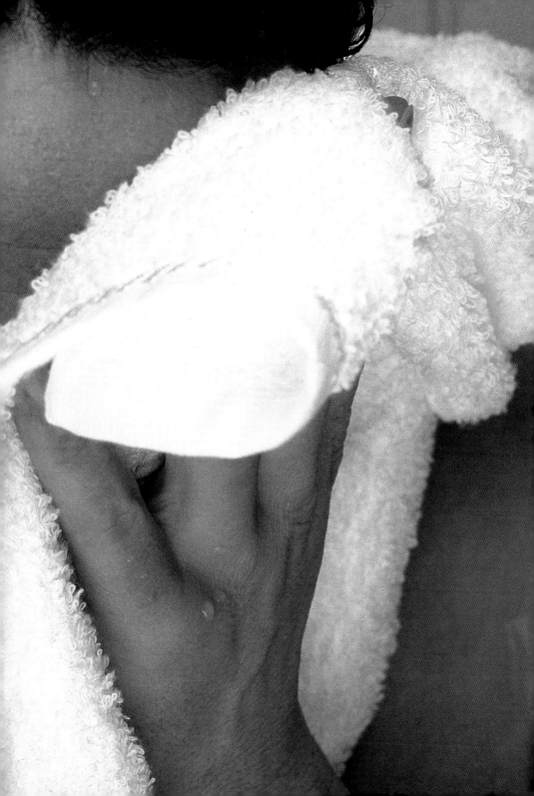

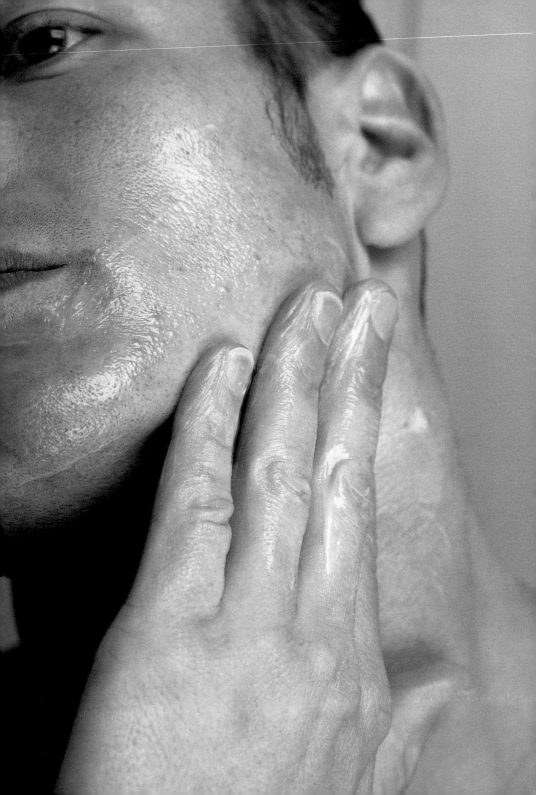

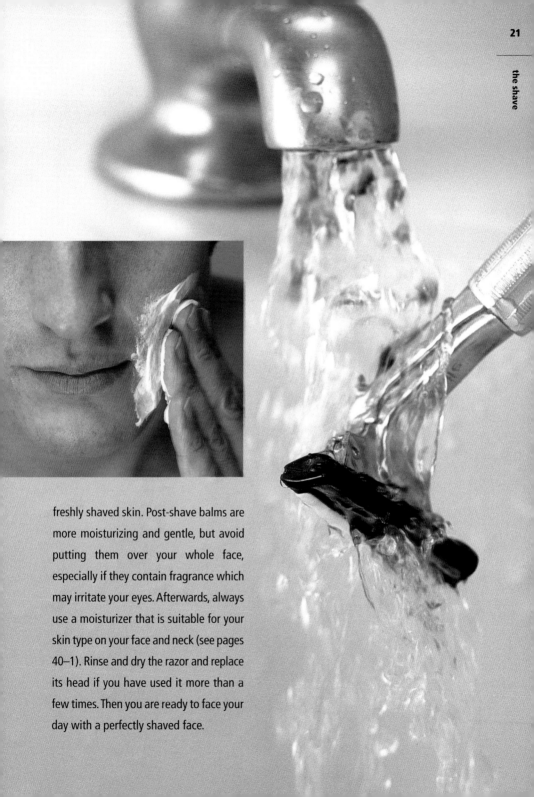

freshly shaved skin. Post-shave balms are more moisturizing and gentle, but avoid putting them over your whole face, especially if they contain fragrance which may irritate your eyes. Afterwards, always use a moisturizer that is suitable for your skin type on your face and neck (see pages 40–1). Rinse and dry the razor and replace its head if you have used it more than a few times. Then you are ready to face your day with a perfectly shaved face.

Electrical case

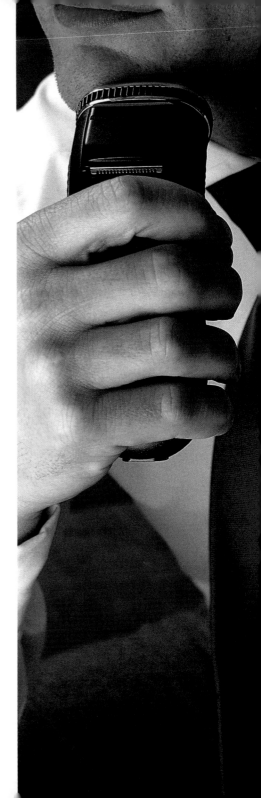

If your idea of a leisurely start to the day is a half-eaten bowl of cornflakes, a shot of strong coffee and a rummage through your drawer for a pair of non-matching socks, using an electric razor is your best bet because you clearly do not have the time to carry out a more elaborate routine. Conveniently, you can even use an electric razor in the office bathroom before your 9 am meeting.

Rotating swivel heads are the most common style of electric razor but they also come in single-headed versions. When the razor is moved slowly over the face, pressed against the skin, facial hairs are removed by protruding through a fine metal mesh that conceals the rotating blades, which then slice off the hairs. The mesh protects your skin from being cut but also prevents the blades from giving as close a shave as a wet razor – your skin will not feel as refreshed and clean as after a wet shave either.

If you are new to electric shaving, your skin may take up to a week to adapt to its new regime and it may feel rougher than usual and even irritated until it has got used to an electric razor. Before beginning your shave, use a pre-electric-shave lotion to lift the beard hairs and prepare your skin.

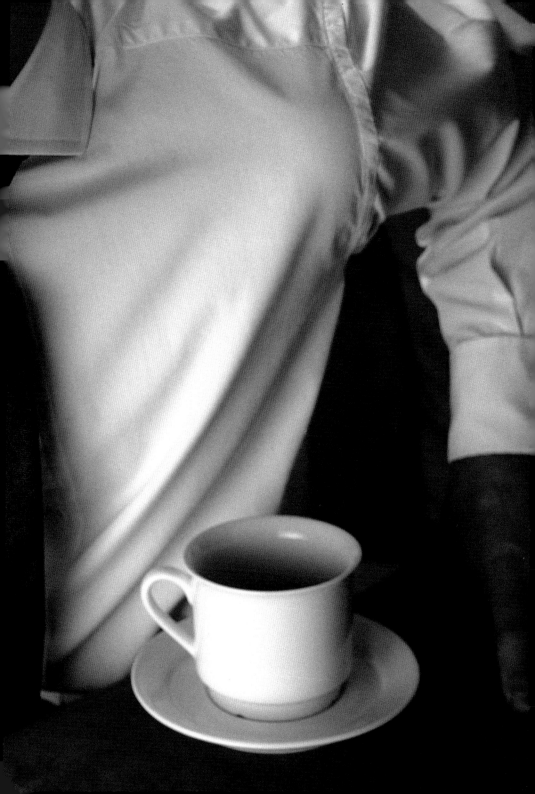

Shaving kit

AFTERSHAVE is alcohol-based and acts as an astringent, which helps avoid infection after shaving and gives a clean fragrance to your freshly shaved skin. Aftershave is the least concentrated form of men's fragrance (see page 100) and can be splashed liberally all over the face and neck. Nowadays, though, many men prefer the more emollient, fragranced shaving balms to a skin-tingling shot of fire water. If you have dry skin you should definitely avoid aftershaves, since the alcohol will dry your skin further. However, for this reason aftershave can be beneficial to oily and acne-prone skins as it helps to eliminate excess oil.

ASTRINGENTS are essentially aftershaves without the smell, and act purely as refreshing, anti-infection splashes for the face. They usually contain alcohol, which will sting, especially if you have cut your skin.

CUTTHROAT RAZORS are sinister implements, which have been around since stubble first sprouted on our chins – originally shells with sharp edges were used as razors by our hairy ancestors. The cutthroat razor, with an ivory handle and unprotected blade, is an elegant but evil-looking relative of the modern razor and is rarely used now, apart from in traditional barber shops. These razors are best avoided unless you are willing to run the risk of more than nicking your skin.

DISPOSABLE RAZORS should only be used in a dire emergency or if you have a very soft beard. With a single head and a lightweight plastic body, they seem determined to cut you no matter how carefully you shave, and if you are used to a double-headed razor the single blade of a disposable razor will feel inefficient and harsh on your skin. Fight with your girlfriend over her bag of disposables as a last resort, and get yourself some new blades fast.

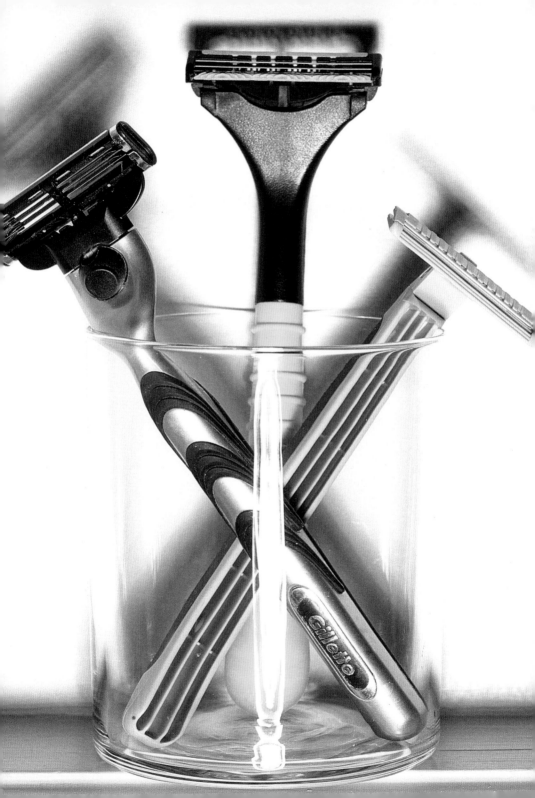

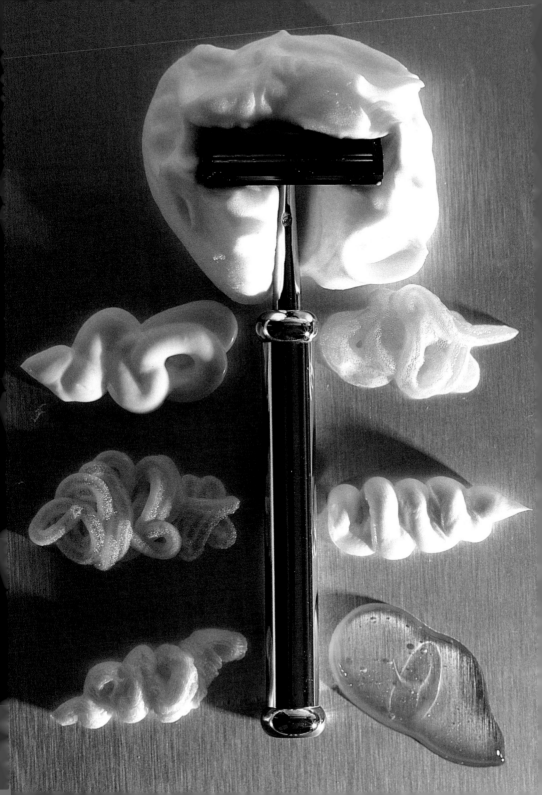

SHAVING BALMS that combine moisturizing qualities together with an astringent have been a boon for men. Many fragrance ranges include shaving balms, so after shaving you can apply an antiseptic, moisturizer and pleasant smell in one simple-to-use product. Only apply these to your beard area, since the fragrance and other ingredients could be an irritant, especially to your eyes.

SHAVING FOAM is a more aerated lubricant than shaving gel. Always shake the can before applying and make sure your beard has been softened and wetted with plenty of hot water. Spray an amount of foam equal to the size of a tennis ball into your hands and then apply it to your face with your fingers. Foam is not as lubricating as gel, but it is fine if your beard growth is not heavy. Try to leave foam on for a few minutes before shaving to make sure your hairs are as lubricated as possible.

SHAVING GEL gets my vote, as it has the consistency of hair gel yet is as slick as a Formula One engine lubricant. A teaspoon of shaving gel should provide sufficient lubrication to remove up to two days' worth of growth. Rub the gel over your fingers to turn it into a dense cream and then apply it to your beard. If you have time, leave the gel on your face for a couple of minutes before starting the shave, as this will soften your beard hairs even more, making them easier for the blade to cut.

SHAVING OIL can give you the closest shave of all when it is used correctly. The oil is usually sold in small 20 ml bottles and only a few drops are needed to lubricate an already wet beard. If your razor starts to drag over your skin during the shave, splash your face with a little more warm water to reactivate the oil. The tiny size of these products means that they are great for travelling, but they can clog your razor quickly, so rinse and tap away the shaved hair from the blade after every couple of strokes.

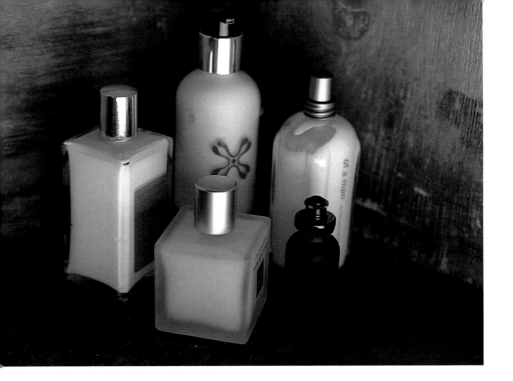

Ingrown hairs

Men with a strong curl in their facial hair, particularly Afro-Caribbean men, may suffer from ingrown hairs, particularly under the chin and around the neck. This condition has a grand medical term, *pseudofolliculitis barbae*. It occurs when the curl of the facial hair is so tight that some hairs do not manage to break through the surface of the skin; instead, they grow back underneath where they are not recognized by the body and are attacked, causing inflammation and infection. Shaving over this area will further aggravate the skin, and the bump caused by the hair can easily be accidentally cut when shaving. John Atchison of the John Atchison Hair Salon, who often treats this condition, advises practising the following:

- Strictly shave in one direction only.
- Do not pull your skin taut to get a closer shave.
- Use a sharp razor with double-edged blades.
- Use tweezers to untangle ingrown hairs, then cut them with your razor or clippers.
- Use an aftershave balm that straightens facial hairs.

Seven rules of successful shaving

1 Do not shave the moment you get up; you will get a closer shave if you wait for at least 20 minutes. This enables your facial muscles to tighten, lifting your whiskers away from your face and making them easier to shave.

2 Soften your whiskers with a hot, damp towel. Wring the towel in hot water and press it over the contours of your face for 20 seconds. It feels great and softens your beard ready for shaving, too.

3 The longer you give your face over to warm water the softer your beard will be, so try shaving in the bath or shower. According to dermatologist Neal Schultz, MD, if you keep the hairs moist, it decreases by two-thirds the force you need to cut them.

4 Wash your face or use a facial scrub (see page 47) before you shave; apart from cleaning your face, the more your beard is in contact with warm water the easier it is to shave. A scrub helps lift the beard from the surface of your skin, enabling the blade to remove it more efficiently. Tip: do not rub too vigorously with a scrub, as it will graze your skin – gentle circular movements of your fingers will do the job better.

5 Go traditional. A shaving brush is a great way of whipping up a beard-lubricating lather. Brushing also helps remove dead skin cells from the surface of your face, ensures that the cream covers every part of the area to be shaved and if you use a circular movement it also lifts the beard away from the face, making it easier to cut.

6 When you have finished shaving use a soft, clean towel to gently pat your face dry; rubbing may irritate your freshly shaved skin and also stretches the skin. Leaving your face slightly damp before applying a shaving balm and moisturizer will help keep the skin of your face hydrated and supple.

7 If your beard growth is especially heavy, apply a moisturizer over your already damp skin before applying your shaving gel – this provides another moisturizing layer, making nicks a thing of the past.

Beards, goatees and moustaches

Fashions change, yet sporting facial hair is probably less popular now than it has ever been. Variations on the goatee (a small beard sculpted close to the chin and around the mouth) are the only acceptable facial furniture (apart from glasses). Yet beards can work as an effective cover-up for scars, acne blemishes and weak chins. And, importantly, some women love them.

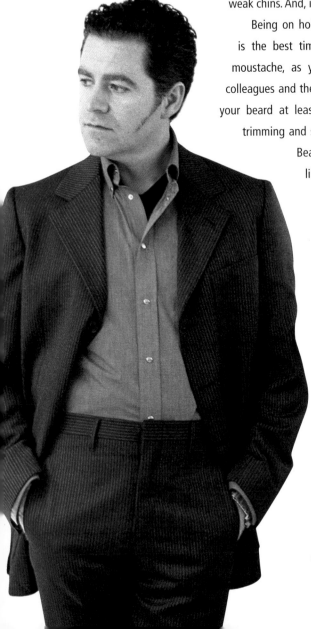

Being on holiday or just being away from work is the best time to experiment with a beard or moustache, as you avoid suffering the ridicule of colleagues and the messy indignity of growing it. Give your beard at least a week to grow and then start trimming and sculpting it into shape with scissors.

Beard or moustache maintenance is a bit like topiary – regular trimming and pruning are a must for a neat result. Let things go and before you know it you will be playing panpipes and wearing a poncho – it is the inevitable result of wearing a bird's nest on your chin.

Here is a guide to beard and moustache shapes and which faces they suit best:

EXTENDED SIDEBURNS that take the form of sharp lines running down the sides of your face parallel to your jaw line, as sported by top hairdresser Charles Worthington (left), accentuate the cheekbones and can give your face extra character.

THE WHIP-THIN MOUSTACHE, as worn by film director John Waters (right), is sharp and sophisticated. It looks dashing, yet a bit dastardly – the look of the cad. It can look rather old-fashioned and eccentric, too; grow it long and wax the ends and you will be a dead ringer for Salvador Dalí.

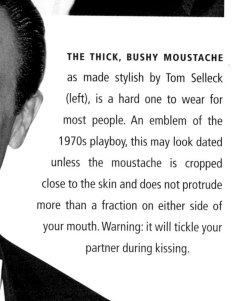

THE THICK, BUSHY MOUSTACHE as made stylish by Tom Selleck (left), is a hard one to wear for most people. An emblem of the 1970s playboy, this may look dated unless the moustache is cropped close to the skin and does not protrude more than a fraction on either side of your mouth. Warning: it will tickle your partner during kissing.

DESIGNER STUBBLE, sported by George Clooney (opposite top), is the classic 1980s-pop-star look, complete with wind-burnt face. If this look suits you, treat yourself to an electric beard trimmer, which will remove a fraction of your beard, leaving the appearance of two or three days' growth. Avoid this look if you have got a job interview, are about to kiss a girl with sensitive skin or intend to wear a jumper (you will end up wearing it on your face). Like beards, stubble can be a good way of covering up acne-scarred skin.

THE FULL GOATEE, including moustache and chin beard, is a high-maintenance piece of facial topiary and requires almost daily trimming. A goatee can look very fashionable, as proven by George Michael (below left).

THE CHIN-ONLY GOATEE – Shaggy's signature chin hair from the cartoon 'Scooby Dooby Doo' – is a hippie-dippy, no-one-understands-me look. This goatee, as worn by Brad Pitt (below), suits a young face and helps emphasize the chin and lower face.

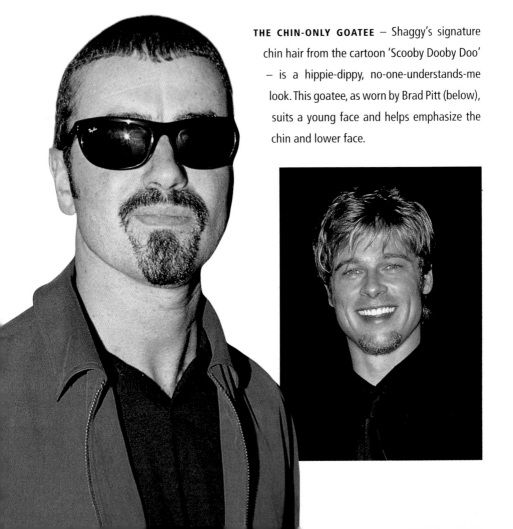

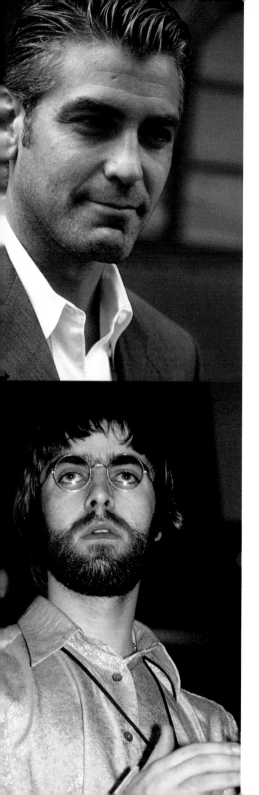

THE FULL BEARD, as modelled by Noel Gallagher (bottom), can look distinguished and vaguely nautical. It can also obscure acne scars and help disguise a narrow face and weak chin.

TOOLS FOR BEARD MAINTENANCE

SCISSORS should be small for intricate snipping – use blunt-ended ones unless you are very confident or a teetotaller, as a wrong move could mean a stabbed nose or worse. Don't let the moustache grow over your upper lip – it will feel like a furry animal trying to climb into your mouth and will become a display for everything you have eaten that day.

CLIPPERS are essential for good stubble maintenance. You can use hair clippers or special beard trimmers, which come with a number of different guards that enable you to vary how much hair is removed. A trim every week should keep things under control, but the rate of growth differs from person to person.

WAXES AND POMADES are old-fashioned but if you want a Dick Dastardly moustache they are the only things that will make it defy gravity. Apply a small amount to your fingertips, rub it through the hair and then twist it into the desired shape.

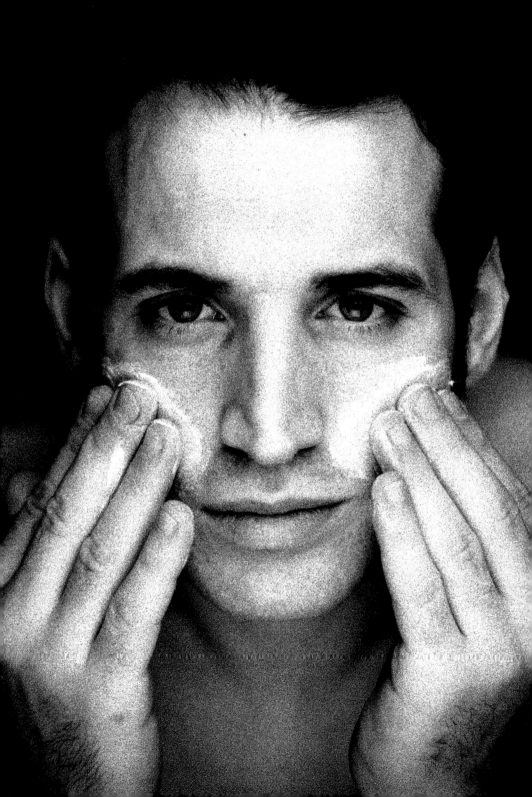

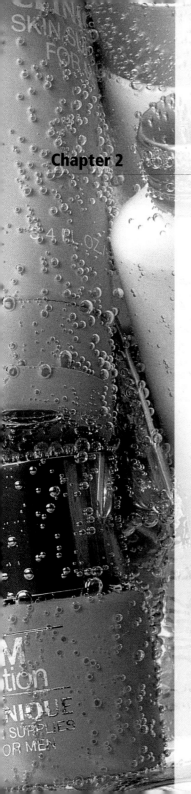

skincare

WHY DO WE SUFFER FROM THE DELUSION THAT THE SPORADIC USE OF SOAP AND WATER AND A SPLASH OF AFTERSHAVE IS ENOUGH TO MAKE WOMEN SWOON, EMPLOYERS FALL OVER THEMSELVES TO HAND US A CONTRACT, AND STRANGERS SMILE AND WAVE WHEN WE WALK DOWN THE STREET? MEN AND SKINCARE ARE NOT TRADITIONALLY HAPPY BED-FELLOWS – MOST OF US GIVE MORE CARE AND ATTENTION TO OUR CARS THAN TO OUR OWN BODIES – YET JUST A LITTLE KNOWLEDGE OF HOW SKIN WORKS AND HOW TO LOOK AFTER IT CAN HELP YOU ACHIEVE CLEAR, HEALTHY SKIN.

YOU WILL SOON REALIZE THAT AHA HAS NOTHING TO DO WITH A DEFUNCT POP GROUP AND EXFOLIATING IS NOT A NEW WAY TO CLEAN YOUR EXHAUST. FOLLOW THE ADVICE ON GOOD SKIN PRACTICE AND YOU WILL FEEL AND NOTICE THE DIFFERENCE IN DAYS, BRINGING BENEFIT TO SURPRISING AREAS OF YOUR LIFE.

what is skin anyway?

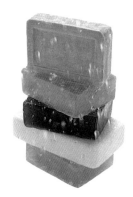

SKIN IS THE **BODY'S LARGEST ORGAN** – it covers an area of about 2 sq m (21 sq ft) and weighs around 3 kg (7 lbs) – and is the barrier between the physical processes of the internal organs and the environment. Skin reduces water loss from the rest of the body and helps maintain a constant body temperature, as well as housing your sense of touch and feel.

Skin is made up of three layers, which are quite distinct from one another yet work together to make your skin a properly functioning organ. The epidermis is the thin, protective top layer, where the cells at the very surface of the skin form the stratum corneum. The dermis, or middle section, is a spongy layer of tissue that supports the epidermis. The subcutaneous layer is the deepest section and is made up of fat cells, blood vessels, glands and bundles of nerve fibres, which feed the skin.

If you woke up one day without your skin you would have instantly lost weight but you would be as vulnerable to the elements as someone taking a stroll to the North Pole wearing no more than a pair of swimming trunks.

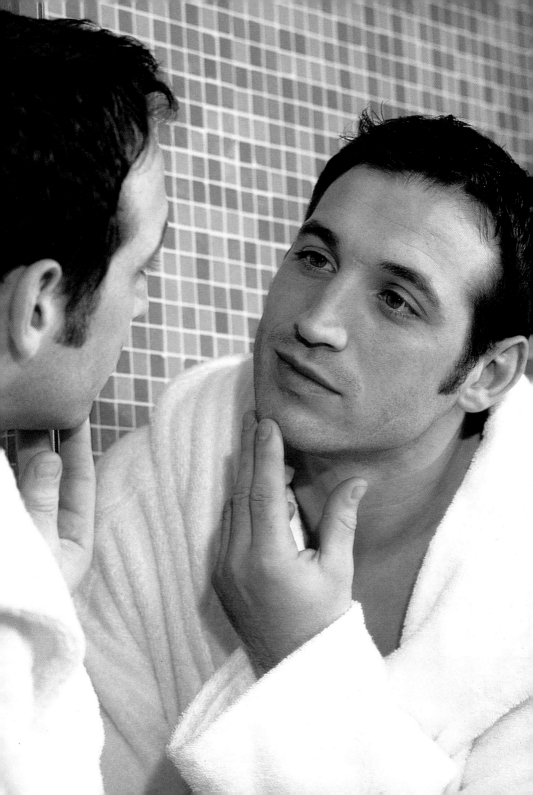

Skin facts

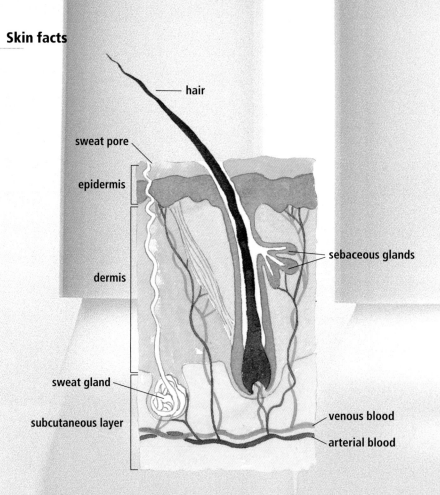

hair

sweat pore

epidermis

sebaceous glands

dermis

sweat gland

subcutaneous layer

venous blood

arterial blood

- All adults have around 300 million skin cells.
- The thickest skin is on the palms of your hands and the soles of your feet and can be up to 4.7 mm (³⁄₁₆ inch) thick. The thinnest is around your eyes and your lips and is only 0.12 mm (less than ¹⁄₆₄ inch) thick.
- A patch of skin measuring 6.5 sq cm (1 sq inch) contains on average 20 hairs, 200 sweat glands, 2 m (6.5 ft) of blood vessels and 30 sebaceous glands.
- Collagen is the elastic property of skin, which slowly reduces as you get older, making the skin wrinkle and sag as its elasticity diminishes. The good news is that men's skin is slightly thicker than women's and contains more collagen, making our skin less prone to wrinkles.

Face facts

Look in a mirror in good light (preferably daylight) before you wash your face and carefully examine your skin. Men's skin is generally more oily than women's because we have bigger sebaceous glands, which are capable of pumping out larger quantities of oil. It may make us shiny, but oil is a natural skin protector and can make us less prone to wrinkling. However, the down side is that oily skin is more likely to suffer from acne and spots. 'Avoid humid conditions,' advises Dr David Fenton, consultant dermatologist at St Thomas's Hospital in London, 'excessive sweating in steam rooms or Turkish baths will aggravate the condition.'

As the body ages the skin goes through various stages of change. During puberty active hormones increase the production of sebum, the skin's natural oil, which is beneficial in moderation. Excess sebum combines with dead surface skin cells and clogs the pores – an uninfected blocked pore becomes a blackhead while an infected one becomes a red spot resulting in a whitehead. To help clear these up, use anti-spot treatments, especially those containing salicylic acid or benzoyl peroxide. During your twenties is probably the best time for your skin, when spots have subsided and the

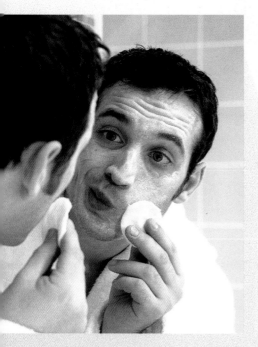

surface is smooth and line-free. As you hit your thirties and forties your skin gradually becomes less efficient at removing dead skin cells, making your complexion look dull (using exfoliants and AHA creams will help brighten the skin and speed up its renewal process). The face also becomes more entrenched with the beginnings of character lines and crow's-feet around the eyes. Into your fifties and beyond your skin will increasingly show the signs of damage caused by exposure to the sun in the form of uneven pigment patches and wrinkling. However, you should still use sunscreen to give your skin a chance to repair some of the earlier damage.

OIL SLICK

If you have greasy skin, your pores, especially around your forehead and nose, will be visible and contain blackheads (small, dark pinpricks of sebum). Your face will look shiny most of the time, except when you have just washed. Oily skin is more likely to suffer from spots than dry skin and is hard to keep looking shine-free. You may feel you have drawn the short straw in the skin lottery, but you have one major benefit – your skin will age better than dry skin. You should use oil-free products on your face and can get away without using a moisturizer at all – but do use sun protection all year round (see pages 56–7). A mildly astringent toner can be effective at combating excessive oiliness, and always keep a clean handkerchief to wipe your nose and forehead before an important meeting or hot date.

DUST STORM

It is hard to see the pores on dry skin, which needs particular care since it is more vulnerable to chapping and flaking. Make sure your face is still slightly damp when applying a moisturizer, as this helps seal in water. Richer creams will be more protective than light lotions. However, do not use products that sit on the surface of your skin – they may be protective, but

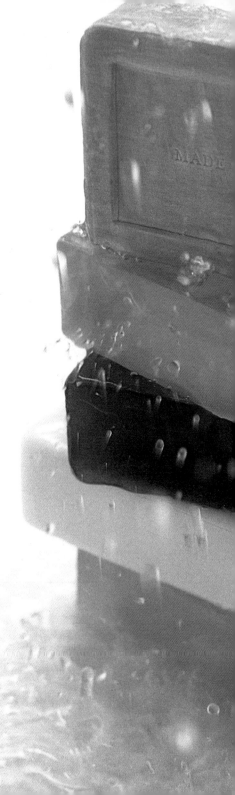

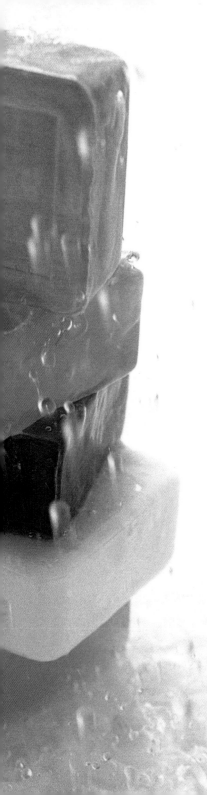

who wants to look greasy? Use a night cream (an especially rich moisturizer) to nourish your skin while you are asleep.

UNITED FRONT

Combination skin, just to make life really complicated, has both oily and dry areas. The T-zone (the middle of the forehead, nose and chin) is greasy with enlarged pores and blackheads, while your cheeks, neck and the rest of your forehead are less oily and tend towards dryness. Avoid putting moisturizer on the oilier parts of your face, but do use it on the drier areas, which still need hydration. To even out the skin, treat the two regions separately in terms of the products you use on them, using oil-based products on the dry areas and oil-free products on the greasy places.

JUST RIGHT

If you have never thought about your skin type and none of the above categories describes your face, then you have normal skin. It is neither excessively dry nor greasy and responds well to basic products that do not need to be overly stripping (to get rid of excess oil) or especially moisturizing (to counteract dryness). You are lucky; this is the best type of skin to have and requires the least maintenance.

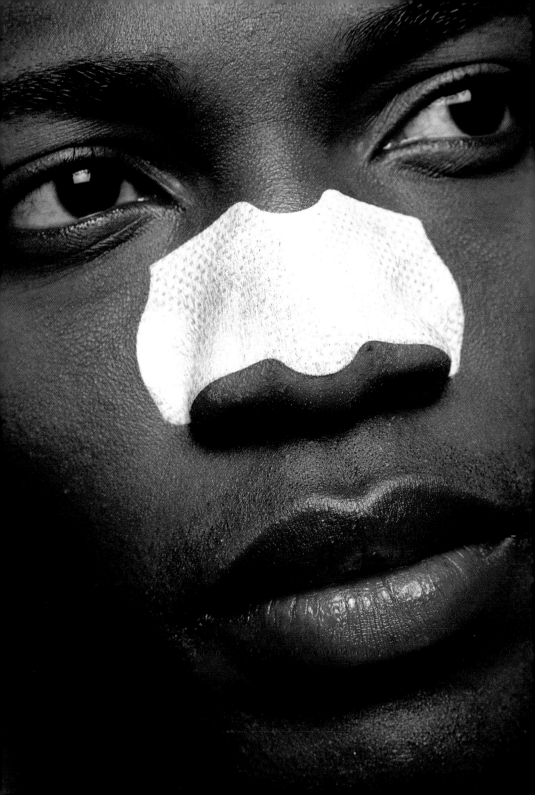

Spot removers

No matter how tempting or whatever your girlfriend says, repeat the phrase: 'I will never squeeze my spots.' Most of us have the occasional break-out caused by stress, lack of sleep or a three-day alcohol binge – so spots are a visible sign of your body telling you to ease up and give yourself a break. Do not attack the culprit by squeezing it with fingers and nails – breaking the skin and spreading the infection will only make matters worse, no matter how satisfying popping the cork might be. The white heads on the top of spots are, in fact, white cells fighting the bacterial infection; they may be unsightly, but they are doing you a favour.

As soon as you notice a big red spot growing on your chin, get hold of some prescription-strength Benzamycin, which combines high doses of zit-busting benzoyl peroxide with antibiotics. This lethal weapon should dry out the culprit in just one night. Less extreme over-the-counter products that contain benzoyl peroxide will have the same effect but will take a few days longer to work. Look out for products containing salicylic acid, which are also effective at giving spots a short shelf life. If you prefer a more natural solution, try ointments that contain tea tree oil, a natural antiseptic, which can also be used on minor cuts, grazes and shaving rash, or just use the essential oil itself, which can be safely applied directly to affected areas.

PULLING THE PLUG

Blackheads are caused by oil from overactive sebaceous glands combining with the debris of dead surface-layer skin cells and plugging up the pores (particularly in the greasy T-zone of forehead, nose and chin where oil glands are especially active). These plugs also stretch the pores, making them look even bigger. Pore strips (self-adhesive strips that grab hold of and pull out pore-clogging debris) are a recent and effective treatment. Apply the strip to wet skin and wait for it to dry (about ten minutes) and then slowly peal it off like a plaster. The strip will be covered in tiny threads of sebum pulled from your pores, leaving your skin smooth, clear and less likely to get blemishes. The only bad news with these miracle workers is that the effects are temporary and may need repeating every week (good news for the manufacturers). Another, even more temporary, quick fix is toner, as it 'shrinks' the pores by slightly swelling the skin around the opening, plumping it up and thus making the pores themselves look smaller.

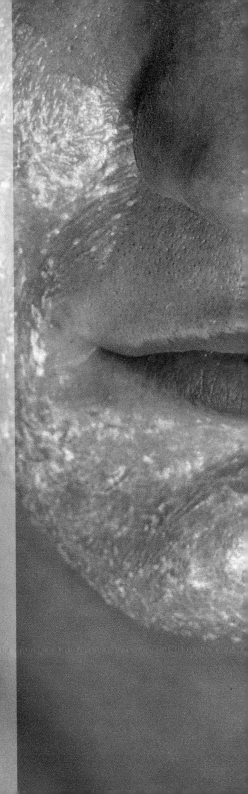

All in a lather

Clean skin helps prevent spots from forming, and freshly exfoliated skin – by removing dead skin cells – further reduces the chance of break-outs and blocked pores. Washing with soap and water is not necessarily the big skincare no-no many people think it is, as long as you thoroughly rinse off any soap residue and never use industrial-strength hand soaps on your face. The tightness in the skin after using soap is caused by a temporary pH imbalance between the soap, which is alkaline, and skin, which is slightly acidic (around pH 6.5). The tightness will ease after about half an hour.

Face washes, either creams or gels, should be used on already-damp skin to create a good lather. Wash with water that is about the same temperature as your body (37.5°C) for the most effective results, and always follow the product's instructions. Many brands have different versions for dry, oily or combination skin types (see pages 40–1), so use a product that is right for your face, morning and night – a non-soap bar is effective on oily skin, while cleansing lotion is more gentle on dry skin. If face washes leave your skin feeling too tight and dry, just use a cleanser in the evening when your skin has accumulated the dirt from your day and rinse with water, or use a facial scrub in the morning before shaving.

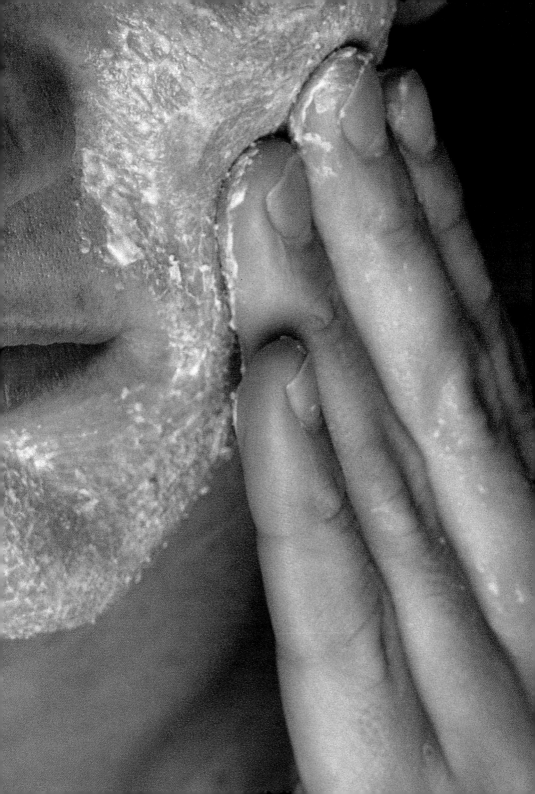

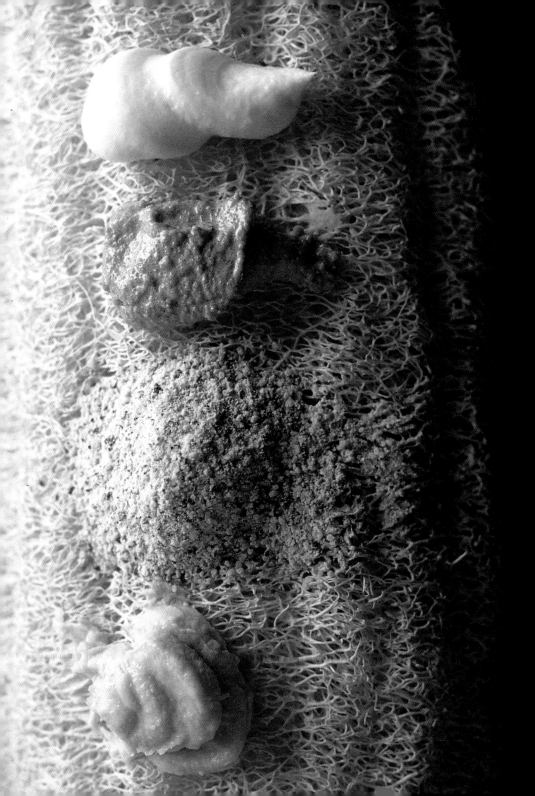

Shedding the old

Using products containing granules is an effective way of sloughing off the surface layer of dead skin cells, which need to be regularly removed in order for the new skin to come though. The granules cause friction, pulling the dead skin away from your face to reveal a glowing complexion underneath. Do not rub too vigorously, however, as scrubs can leave your skin red and sore.

Always follow the instructions on the particular product you are using, but as a general rule a scrub should be used on skin that is already wet. Work the scrub into the skin by moving your fingertips in a gentle circular action. Focus particularly on your chin, forehead and the sides of your nose, where the greasier skin will be building up clogged pores and blackheads.

If your skin is especially sensitive you can apply a scrub and simply leave it on the surface of the skin without rubbing it in, as this will still help remove dead skin cells and promote the renewal process.

Never use a scrub around your eye area, as the skin there is too delicate to take harsh friction. Also, do not use a scrub every day, as it will be too harsh on your skin – once or twice a week should be sufficient.

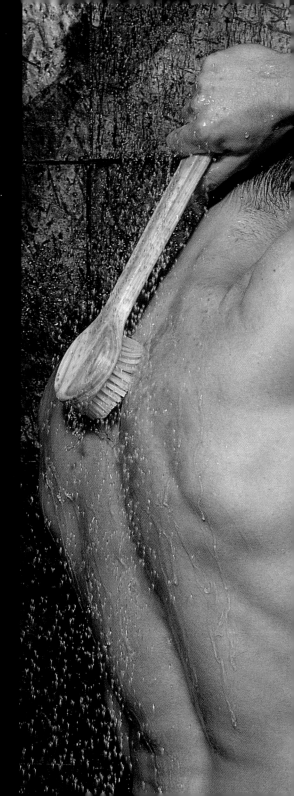

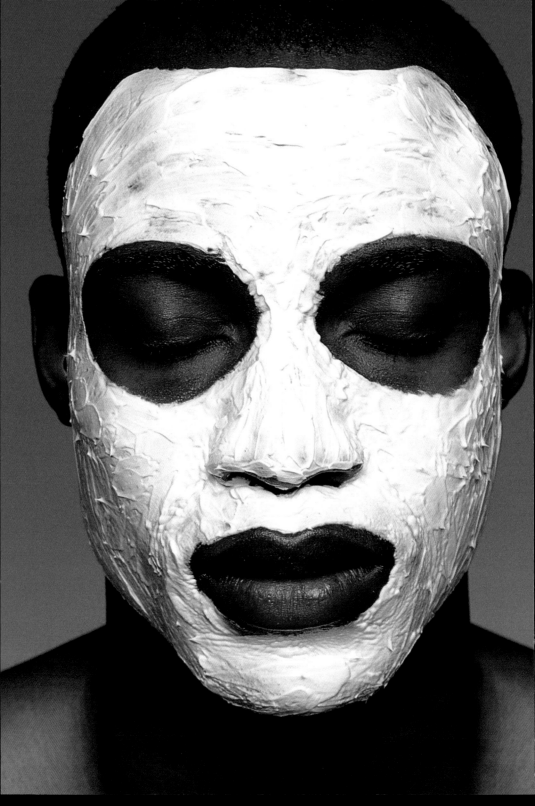

Face masks

There is a mask to suit every skin type and complaint, so make sure you get the most benefit by choosing the right one.

If you have oily skin, go for a mask that contains mud or clay or calls itself 'deep cleansing' or 'clarifying'. These dry to a crust, absorbing debris, oil and dirt from your skin. Do not leave them on for more than ten minutes unless otherwise stated.

Choose a mask that is moisturizing or hydrating if your skin is dry or you have been in a dry atmosphere such as on a plane. These should plump up any fine lines, making your skin look younger.

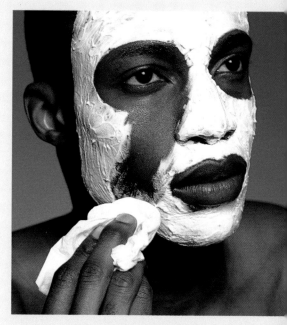

Use a perfecting or replenishing mask if your face is looking tired and grey. These stimulate and boost the skin, and remove the dead surface cells that make your complexion look dull and lifeless.

Gentle, soothing or relaxing masks are for when your skin is red or blotchy and are effective if you have unwittingly spent time unprotected in the sun.

Avoid your eye area when you apply a mask as the ingredients can aggravate the delicate skin. If you have sensitive skin and are using a mask for the first time, do a test patch on your shoulder to see if you have a negative reaction.

Replenishing moisture

Moisturizers are the most commonly used of all skincare products. Every year a fortune is spent on what are essentially simply water- or oil-based creams and lotions. Yet if you have very oily skin you can probably get away without using moisturizer at all, and unless your skin is especially dry you will probably not need to use one when the weather is warm, as your skin will be stimulated to secrete more oil of its own. However, whatever your skin type, do always wear sun protection of at least SPF15. Even the darkest black skins only have a natural protection equivalent to SPF10.

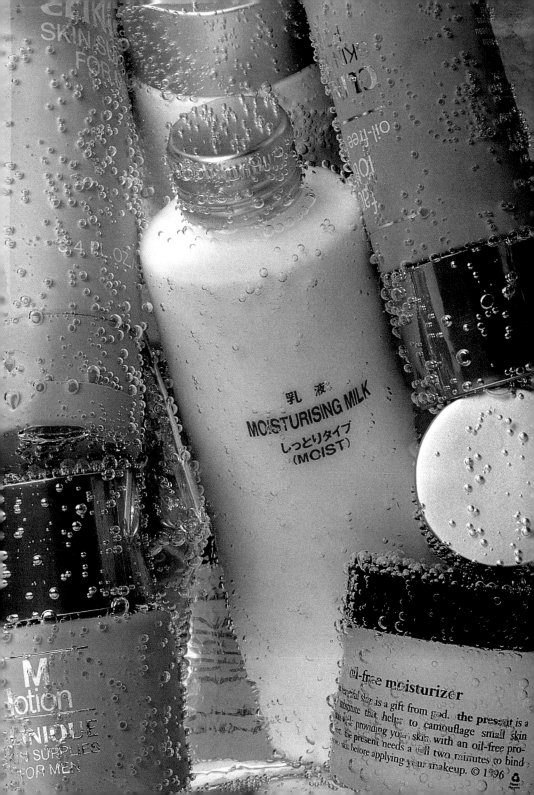

Bottled miracles

The following ingredients are some of the latest breakthroughs in the skincare industry, and are the big guns in the battle against wrinkling and sagging skin associated with ageing. Many of these so-called miracle ingredients are commonly included in cleansers, toners, moisturizers, scrubs and masks.

ALPHA-HYDROXY ACIDS (AHAS) are derived from acids found naturally in fruit and have a brightening effect on the skin. You could rub a slice of grapefruit over your face to get a similar benefit, but you might feel a bit odd. Alternatively, use products with AHAs, which speed up the exfoliation process by breaking down the intercellular 'glue' that bonds dead cells to the skin's surface. These products should be used cautiously, as they can upset sensitive skins and cause redness. If this happens, stop using them or just use them occasionally, maybe once a week.

ANTIOXIDANT VITAMINS A, C AND E are included in some moisturizers and sun protectors to combat the negative effects on your skin of free-radical damage. Free radicals are rogue molecules created through the skin's natural oxidation process, which attack collagen, cell membranes and the skin's lipid layer. Taking these vitamins as supplements in your diet can be beneficial to your skin, too.

BETA-HYDROXY ACIDS are natural acids that are close relations to AHAs and work in a similar way by helping your skin shed its load of dead cells. As with AHAs, irritation can occur, so use them with care.

RETIN-A (also known as tretinoin, retinova and renova) is a compound derived from vitamin A that is an effective form of treatment for acne, sun-damaged skin and wrinkles. Vitamin A compounds help promote cell renewal, slough off dead skin cells and help minimize fine wrinkles. Creams and other preparations containing these compounds should only be used at night, as they react with ultraviolet light and can cause redness and flakiness. For this reason, when you are using skin preparations containing vitamin A derivatives, you should avoid direct sunlight and always wear a high-protection sunscreen (SPF15 or higher).

Eye care

So you have been up all night hitting the bottle or just not getting enough sleep. But getting in late and facing a couple of feminine fists is not what has caused the black circles under your eyes: tiredness has caused them. Also, as you get older the skin around your eyes thins, exposing more bloods vessels near the surface and making the area look darker. Since this thin skin is prone to irritation and lacks active oil glands found elsewhere on the face, it can benefit from soothing eye creams. Free from irritating ingredients, these moisturizers help the skin around your eyes look smoother. The new generation of eye creams also contain light-reflecting particles that bounce light back from the surface of the skin, making your eyes appear brighter and the skin around them paler.

Anything cool and damp applied to closed eyes – such as cotton-wool pads soaked in a gentle toner or water, or even cooled used teabags – will help reduce the puffiness and dark circles associated with tired eyes. For best results, lie down with your feet raised on a pillow for about ten minutes.

The most effective treatment for dark circles, however, is a concealer. This is a skin-toned cream that covers up minor blemishes and uneven skin tone. Before applying a concealer always use an eye cream or moisturizer, as concealers can be drying. Also, use them sparingly: squeeze a pin-head amount of concealer onto the tip of your finger and gently dab, rather than rub, it over the dark under-eye area until you have achieved a natural-looking camouflage. Be careful: concealer is a form of make-up and should be treated with caution. Any hint that you are wearing the stuff is likely to make women run screaming and men give you a wide berth.

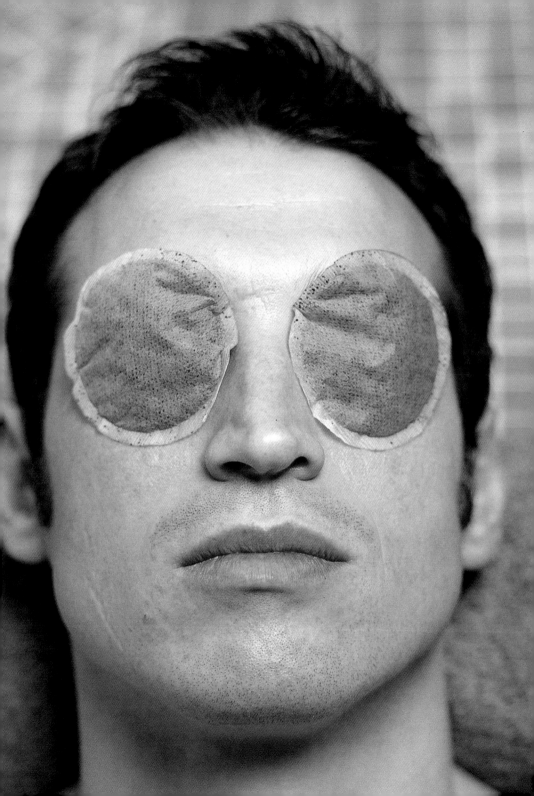

Body works

A couple of times a week before a bath or shower, brush your skin with a body brush, which can be bought from most chemists. A soft-haired brush vigorously swept over your body from your feet upwards and towards your heart helps remove dry skin (especially from your knees, ankles and elbows) and leaves your skin tingling and smooth. Brisk brushing also stimulates the circulation, which speeds up the elimination of toxins.

Even if you have oily skin on your face, the rest of your body could well have a tendency to dryness. To help counteract this, put a teaspoon of olive oil in your bath, especially in hard-water areas where it is difficult to get a good lather with soap. A squeeze of baby oil in the bath is also great for keeping your skin soft. Loofahs, sponges and face cloths used in the bath or shower are good tools for gently removing dead skin build-up from the feet, elbows, knees and hands. As are body scrubs, which have slightly coarser exfoliating particles than face scrubs.

Always follow your bath or shower by applying some body lotion to your still-damp skin, particularly to feet, elbows, knees and hands. It will keep any dry areas of skin smooth and can help avoid the build-up of dead skin, too.

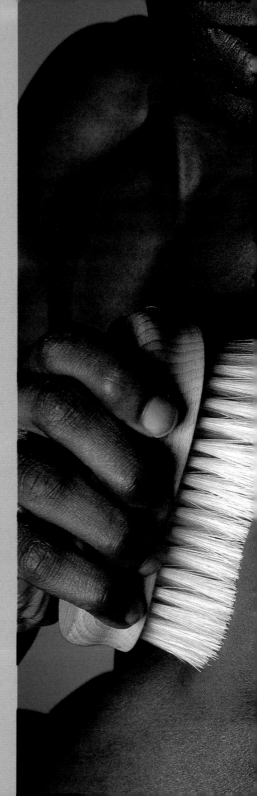

The rules for good skin

Here are four basic rules for maintaining good skin (and health), which even if you do nothing else, are guaranteed to rapidly improve the look and feel of your skin.

1 Drink eight glasses of room-temperature water every day. Drinking water helps the skin perform its vital processes of cell regeneration and renewal – 35 per cent of the body's total water content is found in the skin (see page 132). 'If you are well hydrated all the cells of your body are plumper,' says dermatologist Dr David Fenton. 'Water increases the tension within the cells, but if you are very dehydrated your skin quickly loses its elasticity.'

2 Do not smoke. In addition to the obvious health risks, 'in heavy smokers there is a definite increase in signs of ageing through wrinkling,' says Dr Fenton. 'Smokers have lower levels of vitamin C, which their bodies use up more quickly than non-smokers. Vitamin C applied topically to the skin through preparations can be beneficial and reduces wrinkling.'

3 Eat fresh fruit and vegetables. At least five portions of fruit or vegetables a day are not only the nutritional requirement for good health but for good skin, too. Packed with vitamins and minerals, these foods help keep your skin fresh and glowing (see pages 133–5 for more on good nutrition).

4 No more roasting. Sun and pollution cause the majority of the visible signs of premature ageing (wrinkles to you). So if you want to look like a sheet of crepe paper and risk a dangerous illness, such as a melanoma (the nastiest form of skin cancer), go fry yourself on a beach (see pages 56–7).

Protect and cover

The key to good sunbathing practice is to remember that less is most definitely more – and use your common sense and take the necessary precautions to prevent harm being done. Red, inflamed skin caused by unprotected and prolonged exposure to the sun should be seen as a sign of damage rather than as a prelude to a golden tan. Would you voluntarily scald your skin with boiling water? For the result is pretty much the same when you overexpose your skin to direct sunlight.

The range and quality of suncare preparations has never been so extensive and our knowledge of just how damaging the sun can be is no longer in doubt. Avoiding going out in the sun during the hottest parts of the day (between about eleven in the morning and three in the afternoon when the sun's rays are at their most intense), and arming yourself with a decent-sized bottle of high-protection suncream and a willing partner to help you to apply it (and you to her, too), should keep your skin healthy, as well as prolonging its youthfulness.

Dr David Fenton says: 'People who keep their bodies covered all year round, living in a temperate country, who then spend two weeks overexposing their skin to sun in a far hotter climate, are most at risk from sun damage – their skin just isn't prepared for that onslaught. The big myth is that you look healthier if you have a tan, yet for people who have consistently overexposed their skin to sunlight their skin coloration becomes patchy because of the chronic overstimulation of the pigment cells. Solar keratoses can develop, also known as sun spots, which can then lead to squamous carcinoma or the even nastier melanoma.'

When you are not used to hot weather, it is easy to underestimate the strength of the sun, particularly if there is a cooling breeze or you are by water, which actually reflects the sun's rays and increases the potential damage. When you go on holiday to a hot country always wear a high-factor sun-protection suncream (at least SPF20 at all times – do not work down to lower protection) and reapply it regularly, especially if you are in and out of the water. Try not to go out in the midday sun, wear a hat in direct sunlight and do not feel ashamed to cover up on the beach. Also, drink plenty of water to avoid becoming dehydrated. All of these precautions will give you younger-looking skin for longer, a decreased risk of skin cancer and a smooth, even skin tone. There is no excuse for burning, peeling and generally overdoing it in the sun.

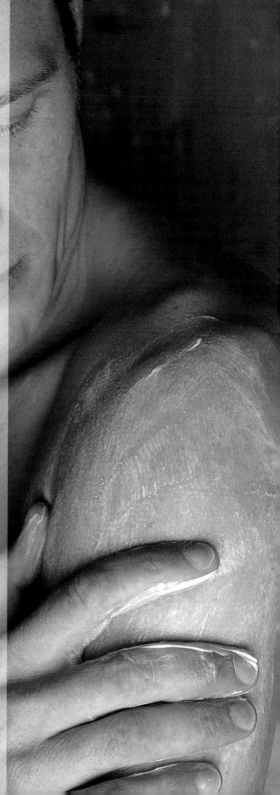

SUN SENSE

1 Apply high-factor sun-protection cream over all your exposed skin before you go into the sun, so you do not get caught out hunting for a good spot on the beach before applying your cream. Get your girlfriend to help you for those hard-to-reach areas like between your shoulder blades – it gives you the perfect excuse to rub some on her, too.

2 Reapply sun protection after every swim in the pool or sea, even if the product you are using claims to be water resistant or waterproof (waterproof sunscreen is the longer-lasting of the two) – if you dry yourself with a towel you will remove the protection. Suncream should be applied every hour in direct sunlight.

3 Avoid lying in the sun during the hottest part of the day (usually between eleven and three) when the sun's rays cause the greatest damage.

4 Always use sunscreen when you go skiing. The combination of altitude and the reflection of sunlight on snow can make skiing potentially more damaging to your skin than towelling yourself with sandpaper. Choose specially formulated suncare products for skiing.

Faking it

Using creams and lotions to fake a tan may seem overly vain, but give them a chance – these products actually work, are safe and, if applied correctly, can create a convincing tan with none of the health risks associated with actual sunbathing. Here are the key points to remember when applying a fake tan.

1   Dry, dead skin will make it hard to get an even tan, so exfoliate your skin first with a body brush, loofah or scrub (do not use anything other than a scrub for exfoliating your face).

2   Thoroughly moisturize the parts of your body you wish to tan, especially dry knees and elbows. This creates a smooth surface on which to apply the tanning products, giving you far smoother, even results.

3   Carefully follow the instructions of the particular product you are using.

4   Only apply the tanning lotion to those areas that would normally tan in the sun – not the soles of your feet.

5   Get a friend to help unless you are a contortionist. How else can you get a tan between your shoulder blades?

6   Make sure your home is warm. You will need to sit around naked or in your underwear until the cream has dried (often as long as a couple of hours). There is one drawback: as the lotion is drying the active ingredients may give off a strange fishy smell and your cat will start licking you. But thankfully, newer products have diminished this smell enormously.

7   Wash your hands and the insides of your wrists thoroughly afterwards. Tanned palms tell the world you have not spent the last month in Hawaii.

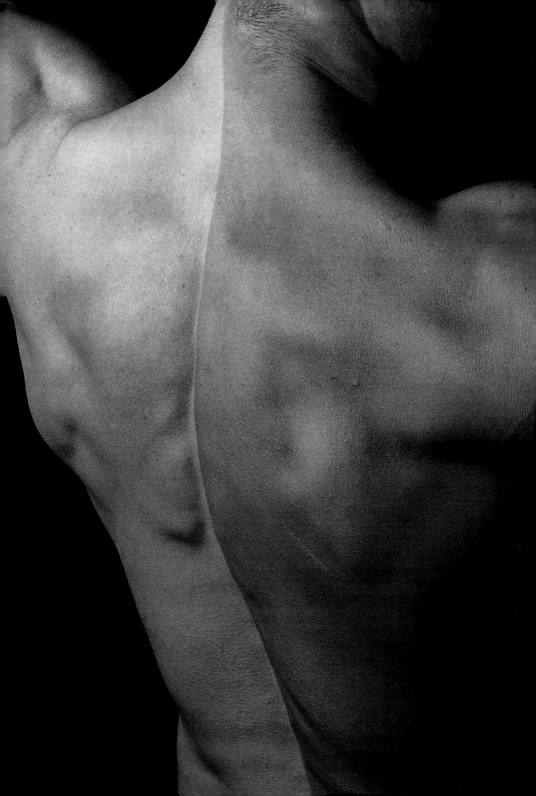

Face Off

If your skin is wrinkled due to sun damage or age, or perhaps your face is scarred by acne, you can choose from a range of medical treatments to resurface and smooth out your skin. Dermabrasion, acid peeling and laser treatments are the key techniques used to remove the top layers of skin (where wrinkles, irregular pigment and scarring reside) in order (when your skin has recovered) to reveal new, unblemished skin. These procedures should only be carried out by a qualified practitioner and full recovery may take several weeks.

ACID TEST Chemical peeling involves painting a caustic solution onto the skin such as glycolic acid, trichloracetic acid or, for extremely scarred or damaged skin, phenol (which removes the most skin). The aim of this procedure is to remove the upper surface of the skin to reveal unscarred, fresh new skin.

RECOVERY After the treatment the skin reddens and needs to be carefully protected before the new skin forms. The new skin is sensitive to ultraviolet light and must be protected with a high-factor suncream.

LIGHT WORKS Pulses of laser light burn off the top layer of skin, tightening it and then removing the damaged upper layers. Some experts claim that laser treatments are more predictable and safer than chemical peels.

RECOVERY Your face will remain pink for a few weeks and should be treated with care and kept out of direct sunlight.

SPIN CYCLE With dermabrasion a dermatologist sloughs off the top layer of skin with a sanding wheel or rotating steel brush. Although it has been practised far longer than the other resurfacing treatments and can seem a bit old-fashioned, dermabrasion is an especially effective technique for removing deep acne scars.

RECOVERY Your face will be raw and will need protective creams, gel dressings and antibiotic medication.

BREACHING THE LINES

Botox is a new treatment that is used to smooth away frown lines and wrinkles caused by the repeated contraction of facial muscles. Those deep furrows in between your eyebrows caused by endless hours spent staring at charts on your computer could be helped by this treatment. The procedure involves a highly purified form of botulin being injected into the facial muscles, which causes the nerve endings to cease to function for three to four months, enabling the lines to lessen and in some cases disappear completely. After a few applications, the treatment seems to be effective for longer, and eventually only one injection a year may be required to stop lines from returning.

Is it safe? The idea of injecting a toxin into muscles to stop them working seems a bit like chopping off your head to get rid of a spot, yet there has – as yet – been no known negative reactions to the treatment. A slight tingling may occur during the injection procedure and the treatment will take a few days to take hold. Surprisingly, the paralysis of the muscles should have no visible effect on your face and you will still be able to pull faces at your boss, petty officials and other irritants.

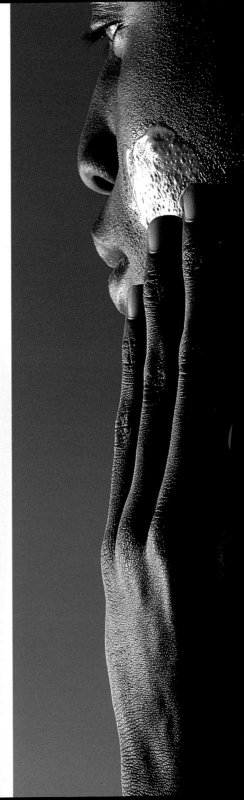

Picture this

Whether you regard tattooing and body piercing as an individual statement or an allegiance to a group or faith, both of these body art forms are becoming increasingly popular. In the USA five per cent of men have some kind of tattoo or piercing.

With tattooing, microscopic punctures are made in the skin with ink to create a permanent picture, words or symbols. The intensity of the ink will slowly fade over time, particularly if the design is exposed to the sun, but it will always remain visible. Removal of tattoos can be costly, painful and lead to permanent scarring. Infrared coagulation is the most advanced tattoo-removing technique, although expect to pay many times the cost of the original tattoo for its removal. Before you commit yourself to a permanent design, why not try out a temporary tattoo – either a transfer, mehndi (henna paste) or body paint? Warning: never tattoo your girlfriend's name on your body, as its removal could be more painful than any emotional break-up.

Piercing is a puncture wound and some areas like the ears and tongue heal within weeks while the navel and nose can take months. If the equipment used is not sterilized

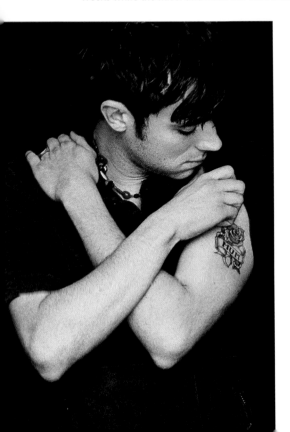

piercing can result in a nasty infection; it can also be a fairly painful experience.

Before you embark on either procedure your primary concern is for your safety. Only use practitioners who have been recommended to you and adhere to high standards of hygiene – check that they only use sterilized materials and single-use tools. This will prevent the transmission of blood-borne pathogens like hepatitis B and C and HIV (the AIDS-causing virus).

For many fans of body art, the first time is just the beginning of a long journey into self-expression. One tattoo or piercing was clearly not enough for Lenny Kravitz (opposite), and Damon Alban (left) has begun the process – but where will it end?

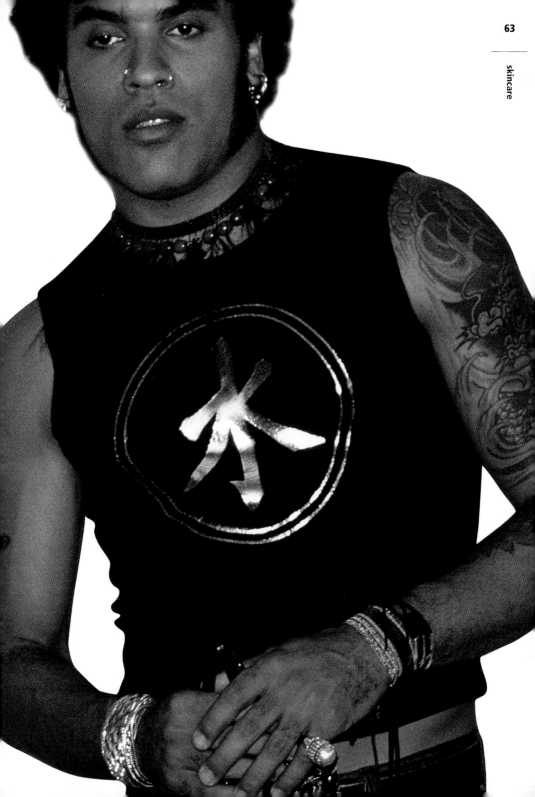

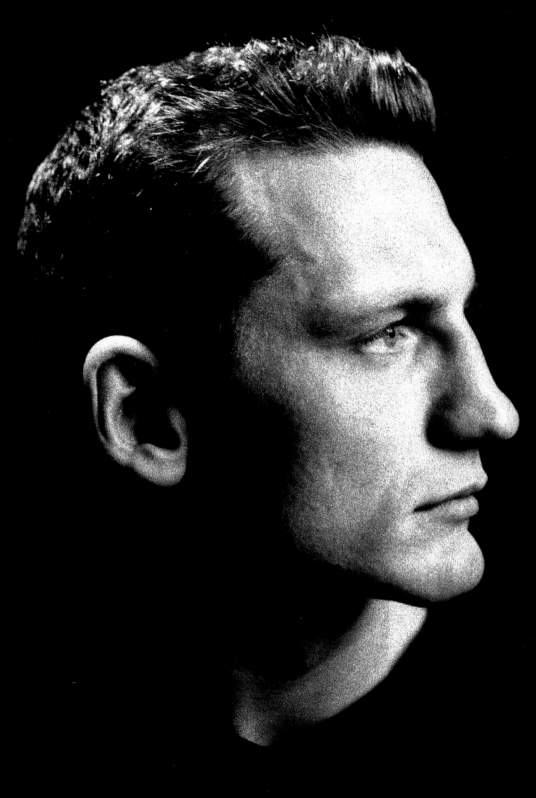

haircare

WE COME INTO THE WORLD BALD AND WILL PROBABLY LEAVE BALD, AND IN BETWEEN IS A WORLD OF SHAMPOOING, CONDITIONING, TRIMMING, RESTYLING, DYEING, BLOW-DRYING, TWEAKING, COMBING, BRUSHING AND COAXING. HAIR IS A FULL-TIME JOB, AS LONG AS YOU HAVE GOT SOME TO PLAY WITH.

AN AMALGAM OF KERATIN (PROTEIN) AND MELANIN (PIGMENT), HAIR IS THE CAUSE OF SO MUCH ANXIETY AND HARD WORK BECAUSE IT IS A POTENT (AND VERY VISIBLE) SYMBOL OF WHO WE ARE AND HOW WE SEE OURSELVES. LONG LOCKS ARE A SIGN OF INDIVIDUALITY AND ABANDON (THINK HIPPIE, SURFER DUDE OR AGEING ROCK STAR), WHILE NEAT CROPS, SPORTED BY MONKS AND THE MILITARY, IMPLY CONFORMITY AND DISCIPLINE. PROFESSIONAL MEN FALL INTO THE LATTER GROUP AND NEED SHORTER STYLES, CUT TO SUIT THEIR FACE AND HAIR TYPE.

healthy, shiny hair

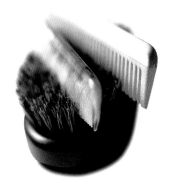

THE SHINE GIVEN OFF BY **HEALTHY HAIR** is created by the scales that encase the hair shaft lying flat and smooth. Each individual hair has an oil-secreting gland attached to the hair follicle at the base, which helps to keep the scales smooth and even. When a mass of hairs lie together uniformly, reflecting light off each strand, the whole head of hair will look lustrous and healthy.

Maximizing the shine of your hair is the main goal of good haircare and your enemies in the battle for a great head of hair (including hair loss, of course) are primarily pollution, chlorine, overheating and bad brushing technique. Haircare companies attempt to improve on nature by providing your hair with oils and proteins to enhance its shine. Overdo this process and you will end up having to use a clarifying shampoo to clear away all the build-up before starting the process once again.

Washing your hair once a day or every other day is fine, but use a gentle, frequent-wash shampoo so that your hair is not stripped of its natural oils, making it look dull and dry. If you style your hair with a dressing, such as wax, gel or pomade you may not need to use conditioner since the hair shafts will have some protection from the dressing.

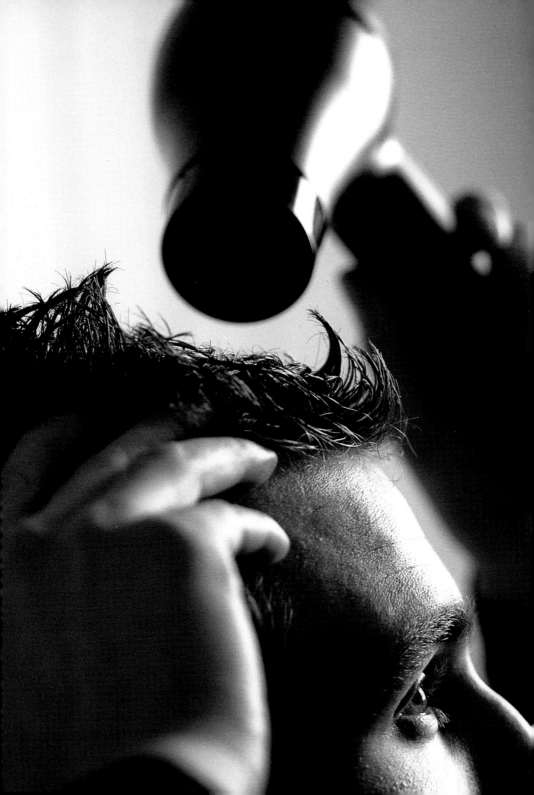

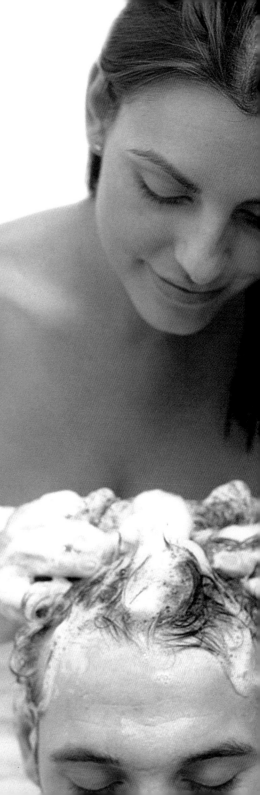

The three rules of good haircare

1 Regularly wash your hair with a mild shampoo – even every day unless your scalp is overly dry; if it is, wash it every other day and rinse and massage your scalp on the non-shampoo days. Avoid the overuse of anti-dandruff shampoos, which can turn your hair into wire wool. Only use them when you have a scaly break-out and switch back to a regular shampoo once the flakiness is alleviated. Regardless of dandruff, alternate two or three different brands every few months to avoid the build-up on your hair caused by constantly using the same product.

2 Use a conditioner that smooths and thickens your hair and increases its shine and bounce. As with shampoo, find one that suits your hair type (oily, normal or dry) and leave it on for a few minutes before rinsing. Leave-in conditioners are also a good idea, especially if you have very dry hair or are inclined to get carried away with the blow-dryer.

3 Dry your hair carefully. After washing your hair, towel dry it and then leave it to dry naturally, or blow-dry it on a medium to high heat with the weakest air-flow setting. Do not overdry your hair; leave it slightly damp to avoid damaging it.

Know your products

CLARIFYING SHAMPOO should be used occasionally – usually once a month is sufficient – to clean away the build-up of other hair products, which can stay on the hair shaft, making your hair look dull.

CONDITIONER is a post-shampoo cream applied to wet hair and then rinsed out. Conditioner adds vitamins, moisturizer, shine, protein and de-tangler to your hair. Leave-in versions are good for damaged or overheated hair.

GEL makes hair easier to style and holds it in place; it is particularly good for styling short hair. If you put it on wet hair, it dries hard and creates a wet look; on dry hair, it eliminates flyaway strands, keeping your locks under control. A teaspoon of gel should be enough for shorter styles.

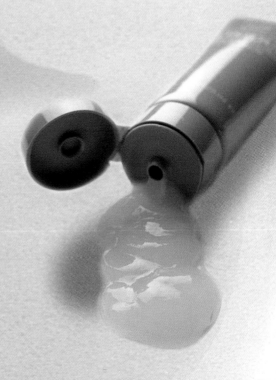

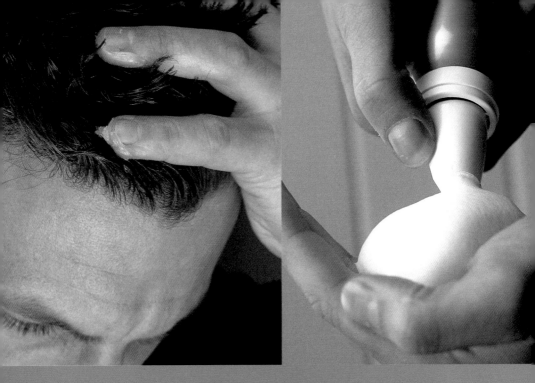

GLOSSER, SHINER, POLISHER AND LAMINATOR are all names that describe a lotion or cream containing large amounts of silicone or oil, which you rub onto your hair to smooth it, tame curls and frizz, and make it gleam. Just a few drops should be sufficient – overdo it and you will end up looking like an oil slick; less is usually more with these products.

MOISTURIZING PRODUCT is a term used to describe any shampoo, conditioner and treatment that softens dry or coarse hair. Many contain glycerine, which helps hair capture and retain moisture.

MOUSSE is a foaming conditioner that helps hold hair in place. A little mousse expands onto your hand to about the size of a tennis ball; rub it through wet hair and then dry to give control and body. Mousse is especially good for controlling longer, wavy hair.

SPRITZ OR SPRAY GEL is a light, liquefied gel, which is applied as a mist to keep hair in place. Good for all hair textures, spray gel can be applied to wet or dry hair.

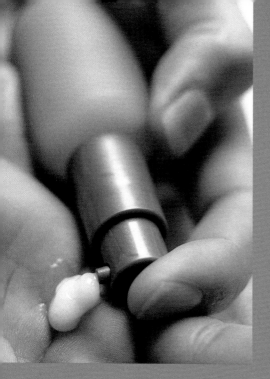

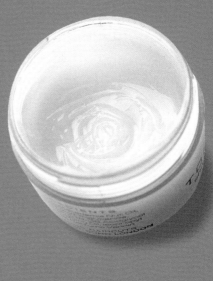

THICKENERS, VOLUMIZERS AND BODY BUILDERS are ingredients that are found in most shampoos and conditioners, and are also available as stand-alone products. They either infuse hair with proteins or coat it with polymers or waxes to make it seem thicker and fuller. These products can be especially effective at creating the illusion of volume on fine or thinning hair.

WAX AND BRILLIANTINE are heavy oil-based hair dressings. The idea of them may seem rather old-fashioned but these products are effective at giving texture, shine and hold to shorter hair styles. Apply small amounts of wax at a time, building it up gradually until you get the desired degree of hold and texture. If you apply too much, you will have to shampoo it off and start again. Gentle shampoos may find it a struggle to get these products completely out of your hair, so go for special heavy-duty versions that are formulated to remove all traces of hair wax without stripping the hair of its natural oils. Another effective method for removing wax is to use neat shampoo on your head before adding water – just rub the shampoo thoroughly through the hair, then wet it, rinse as normal and repeat.

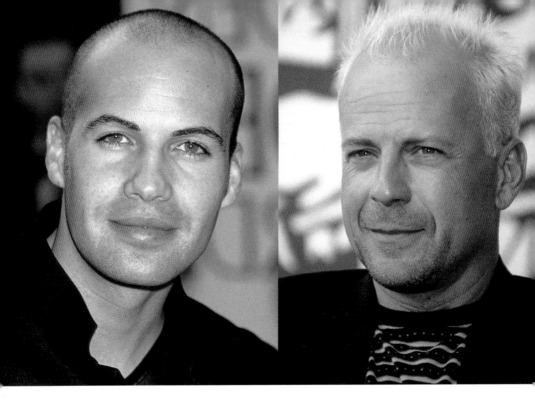

Losing your hair; what should you do?

It was clearly a bald man who asserted that men who are thin on top are more virile than their hirsute brothers. Yet balding men go through an agony of self-consciousness and resort to bizarre and often dangerously unscientific remedies to stem hair loss. Far better to accept the change, keep your hair short and fall in love with the shape of your head.

A CUT ABOVE THE REST

If you have lost more than a third of your hair, go for the shortest style you feel comfortable with. 'Hormones are the reason for hair loss,' says Daniel Hersheson, a London hair-dresser and haircare expert. 'If you are balding, the best advice I can give is do not try to hide it; have your hair cut very short, and keep it neat with a little cream or wax. Billy Zane (above left), Bruce Willis (above right) and Anthony Edwards (opposite) all do.' Growing facial hair is a good way of detracting from the hair loss on your head. Most importantly, never try to hide your baldness by scraping long strands over it from other, more thickly covered parts of your head. It never looks good and will merely emphasize your baldness.

DRASTIC MEASURES

Hair replacement surgery can be painful and expensive (prices start from around £3,000/$4,800), although modern micrografting technology (pinpricks to you) has come a long way since hair was grafted in fake-looking chunks. Now single hairs are transplanted and placed at the natural angles of usual hair growth. 'When it is done properly, nobody will ever know,' says Dr Dominic Brandy, who carries out the procedure at his practice in Pittsburgh. Although Dr Sheldon Kabaker, MD, associate clinical professor at the University of California, San Francisco, says that the treatment can have some side effects, including scarring. His best advice is to thoroughly check out the reputation of any surgeon you approach and be wary if he or she has not been practising in the area for long.

A SMALL WIG

If surgery is too expensive an option to consider, a less invasive alternative is to wear a toupee (stop sniggering at the back). Like surgery, things have moved along mightily in hair technology, making a custom-made toupee polybonded into place an acceptable alternative to a bald pate. Toupees are now so good you can even shower while wearing one. If you wear a hairpiece, the key to its success is to be relaxed about it; feel self-conscious and people will instantly be able to tell that you are actually wearing a real-hair hat.

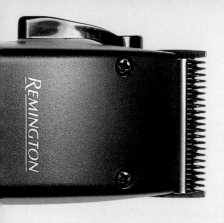

HOPE IN A BOTTLE

Minoxidil is a chemical marketed under a variety of brand names in the treatment of hair loss. It does have extensive scientific backup for its efficacy, but it is not a cure for baldness. Minoxidil slows down the rate of hair loss but cannot replace hair that has already gone. Also, its chances of success are far better for men who have only been losing hair for five years or less, and its long-term success has yet to be fully discovered. Expect to pay around £25/$40 (for 60 ml) a month and remember that results only last while you continue to use the product.

Prepecia is hailed as a new wonder drug in the fight against hair loss, but currently it is only available in the USA. It blocks the conversion of testosterone into follicle-shrinking DHT (dihydrotestosterone, the hormone that causes male pattern baldness). A study by the American Academy of Dermatology in New York found that 86 per cent of users had no further hair loss while popping the pills. However, four per cent suffered a loss of sex drive.

Which hairstyles will suit me?

'The key to getting the right haircut is all about balance,' says Marlene Vendittuoli, specialist in men's grooming at DJ Rubin Salon in New York. 'You want to counteract the shape of your face by choosing an opposing shape for your hair.'

If you have a narrow face go for more volume of hair at the sides of your face, as David Bowie has (left), sporting a near-perfect example of a flattering haircut for a narrow face. Ask your stylist to cut your hair very close at the ears, then gradually add length up past your temples, but keep it fairly short on top. The overall effect will add volume to the sides of your face, instead of more length. 'Anything that is too long on top will accentuate the length of your face, and that is something you want to avoid,' says Damien Miano, of Miano-Viel Salon and Spa in New York.

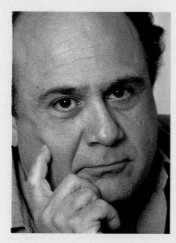

If you have a round face, balance out the roundness by having a haircut with straight lines. Ask your barber or stylist to taper the hair very close at the sides and, as the head gradually rounds, leave a little more length on top, creating a square shape. If you have this face shape and thinning hair, have it cut even closer to your head, as length at the sides will only accentuate the lack of hair on top. With a high, domed forehead and round face, Danny De Vito (left) is wise to keep his hair short.

'Men with square faces are the most fortunate,' according to Miano. 'They can pull off virtually any hairstyle.' The floppy locks of Matt Damon (below) only seem to enhance and flatter his regular features and face shape. The only thing to avoid is a square cut on a square head, unless you wish to resemble Frankenstein. When you get your hair cut, just say: 'Long on top, full on the sides, but give it some proportion.' If your hair is thinning, be sure that it gets gradually shorter from the top of the head downwards. Medium-length sideburns are best – they accentuate your jaw without overdoing it.

BARBERS OR HAIRDRESSERS?

If you have a short cut that need trimming every two or three weeks, a traditional barber could save you a lot of money. You will not be pampered or get a cutting-edge style, but you should be out in under half an hour with a neat, classic cut. If you wear your hair longer, use colour or want a more fashionable style, go to a salon and be prepared to pay more. You will have a consultation with a stylist about which cut will suit you, and for personal treatment salons are far superior to barbers. To keep your hair in good condition a cut every four to six weeks should be sufficient.

Dyeing your hair

Colouring your hair can help cover up grey hairs and add lustre to your locks, giving your hair noticeable life and depth. Hair colour expert Daniel Galvin advises the following: 'When dyeing your hair it is best to choose a colour that is two shades lighter than your natural hair colour – this will almost definitely be the right choice for you. Your skin tone and the colour of your eyes should also be taken into account.' Galvin also suggests trying highlights or lowlights (lightening or darkening small strands or even slices of your hair) as an effective way of 'softening a man's haircut, which can often be very short and solid in colour.'

If you are beginning to go grey, do not despair. Bear in mind that grey hair can look very distinguished (think Richard Gere, Paul Newman and Kris Kristofferson), and is far less disturbing for men than losing their hair. 'Grey hair is a collection of grey, white and silver natural highlights,' says Daniel Galvin. 'Men can colour their hair to tone down the white to one or two shades lighter than their natural colour.' There are now many good products on the market for men to colour their greying hair at home, but it is advisable to experiment on just a small section of hair to be sure you have found the one that suits you best before committing yourself to it. And, as always, make sure you follow the product's instructions carefully.

If grey hair is not a worry for you – yet – but you fancy trying out a new look without going to the hassle and expense of having a permanent colour change done in a salon, there is a raft of over-the-counter products available to help you change the colour of your hair to great effect. Chemical dyes come in three types – semi-permanent, which last for six to eight shampoos; longer-lasting versions, which last for up to 20 shampoos; and permanent dyes, which will last as long as two to three months. Alternatively, you can just use a very temporary colour, which can be easily washed in with a special shampoo or applied through a mousse or gel. Henna is one such example and is a vegetable dye, which, rather than penetrating the hair shaft, coats the outside of it with colour, usually giving a semi-permanent reddish tint to the hair that is brighter when you first apply it and gradually becomes more subtle after a few washes. Chemical colours contain ammonia and peroxide, which are able to penetrate the hair shaft, and although they sound quite dramatic, most modern products are surprisingly gentle on the hair and do not hugely affect its condition.

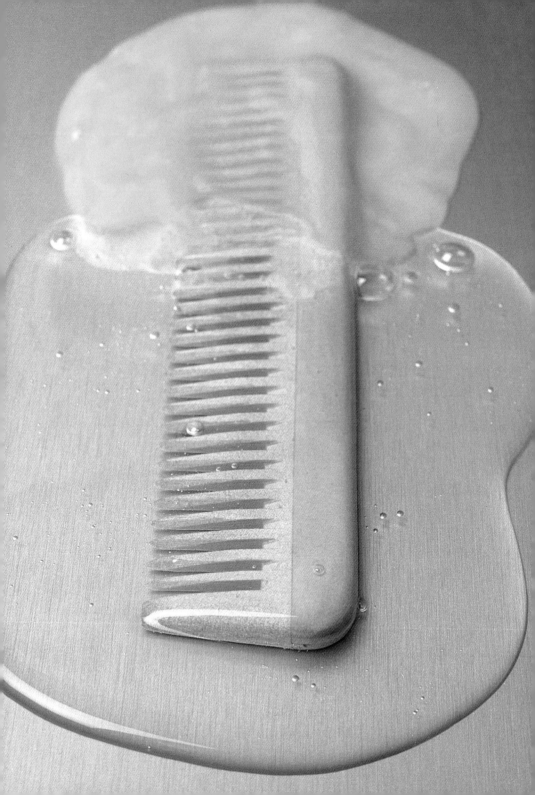

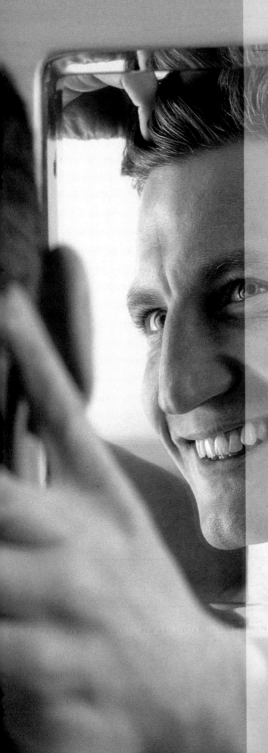

Dandruff

Almost everyone suffers from a flaky scalp occasionally. Your scalp dries, you itch, small bits of dead skin fall off: that's scalps for you. It is not very pretty, but fortunately clothes brushes do exist. However, at some time or another 20 per cent of the population will suffer from dandruff (also known as seborrhoeic dermatitis), which is caused by the yeast *pityrosporon ovale*. If you do suffer from this condition it will be some relief to know that you are certainly not alone and it is easy to treat.

'The basic remedy for curing dandruff is fairly simple,' assures Dr Jacobson, a trichologist from the Balor Hair Research and Treatment Center in the USA. 'Use an anti-dandruff shampoo that suppresses the yeast's activity on your scalp. The active ingredient you are looking for is selenium sulphide. Make sure you follow the instructions on the bottle and expect the treatment to take two or three weeks to be effective.'

TAKE A SPIN Another procedure that may help is to rotate shampoos, since sometimes your hair and scalp build up a kind of immunity to the same shampoo used daily. Rotate several anti-dandruff shampoos for better results.

TRIM OUT STRESS Several conditions that commonly cause dandruff are all influenced or aggravated by stress. Just knowing that dandruff may be related to stressful situations in your life may lessen your worry about what is causing the dandruff and eventually clear up the flaky problem.

SHED SOME SUNLIGHT Sunlight may actually temper the growth of the yeast, according to some dermatologists.

RAID THE LARDER Dr Shupack, professor of clinical dermatology at New York University Medical Center, recommends massaging a few drops of olive oil into your scalp after shampooing at night, covering your head with a shower cap and shampooing again in the morning.

CHEMISTRY LESSON Non-prescription hydrocortisone lotion relieves the inflammation that leads to dandruff – a stronger prescription cream is also available. For stubborn cases, resort to ketoconazole, which is found in prescription antifungal shampoos. Over-the-counter treatments rarely fail to rid scalps of dandruff, but in exceptional cases a referral to a dermatologist will enable more concentrated products to be prescribed.

DANIEL HERSHESON'S TOP TIPS FOR A GREAT HEAD OF HAIR

1 Have your hair cut regularly (at least once a month) to maintain the style and keep it in good condition.

2 Use a good-quality shampoo that is designed for your specific hair type (dry, greasy or prone to dandruff).

3 Wear your hair to suit your lifestyle – do not keep your hair long and in your eyes if you are very active or your job is manually intensive.

4 Change your style with fashion or you will never look any different.

5 If you use a gel or some other styling products, use a clarifying shampoo every three or four weeks to get rid of any build-up, or your hair will soon become difficult to style.

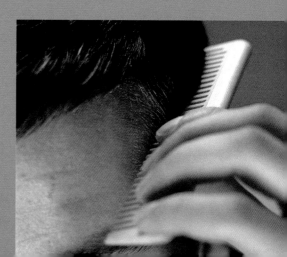

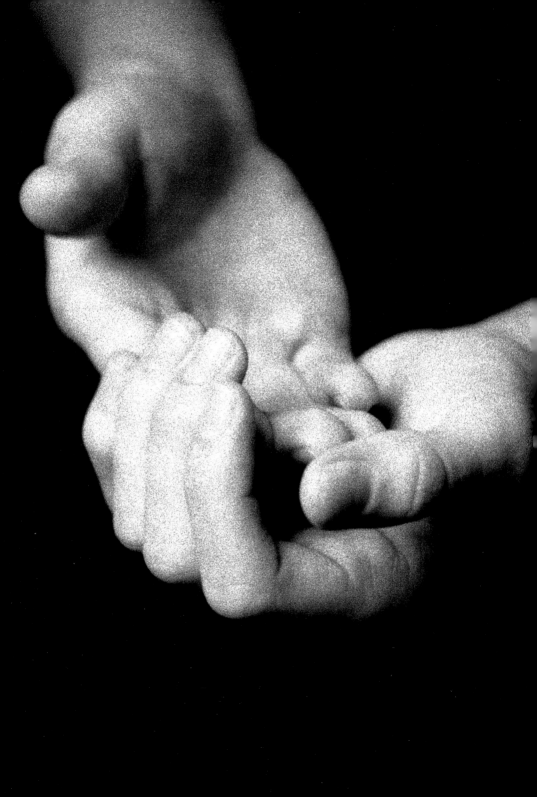

Chapter 4

fine tuning

REMEMBER BEING TOLD AT SCHOOL HOW TO PRESENT YOURSELF FOR A JOB INTERVIEW? CLEAN SHOES AND NAILS WAS ABOUT THE SUM OF IT; NOT FORGETTING THE DARK, SOBER SUIT AND A WINNING SMILE. THE ADVICE HAS NOT CHANGED MUCH, ALTHOUGH IT IS PROBABLY BEST TO LEAVE THE BLACK TIE AT HOME SO YOU DON'T LOOK LIKE YOU ARE GOING TO A FUNERAL. IF YOU TURN UP ON THE BIG DAY LOOKING UNGROOMED AND UNKEMPT, YOU ARE ADVERTISING THE FACT THAT YOU ARE A LOW-DOWN REPROBATE BEFORE YOU HAVE EVEN SHOWN YOUR GREYING TEETH.

WHEN IT COMES TO GIVING A GOOD IMPRESSION IT IS OBVIOUSLY THE VISIBLE PARTS OF YOURSELF THAT NEED THE MOST ATTENTION, BUT DO NOT NEGLECT OTHER AREAS OF YOUR BODY THAT ARE NOT ALWAYS ON DISPLAY – YOU NEVER KNOW WHEN YOU MIGHT BE CALLED UPON TO EXPOSE YOUR FEET.

attention to detail

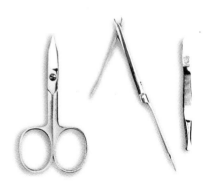

GOOD GROOMING IS **ALL ABOUT PERFECTING** the fine details of your appearance, so that whatever you may do to prove or disprove people's first impression at a later date, it will always start off as positive. Excess hair on your face where there shouldn't be any, ragged fingernails, gnarled feet, yellow teeth and less-than-pleasant breath are bound to be held against you. A bit like dressing well – you might just be wearing jeans and a T-shirt but the right footwear or a decent watch can make you look stylish even at your most casual – if you keep the details under scrutiny you should always look neat.

Whatever happens to the hair on your scalp, your body will become more hairy as you age. You may be wearing all the right clobber – Savile Row suit, Italian loafers, silk tie – but if you have got hair curling out of your nostrils you might as well be wearing a badge saying, 'Slob'; the hairs are all people will see. A few simple tools and a well-lit mirror are all you need to improve your chances of being considered a well-groomed man. Also essential is the ability to sustain a few pinpricks of pain – plucking is not the same as shaving, after all. You are not aiming to get an arched eyebrow to rival your girlfriend's or remove all your nasal hair (necessary to filter airborne debris), just to keep everything under control.

Hairy monsters

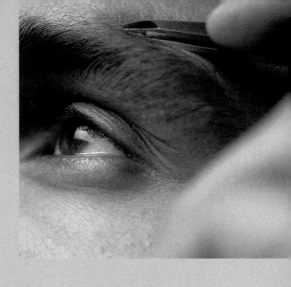

As your body hair becomes more fertile, your eyebrows may decide to meet in the middle of your brow and shake hands, creating a monobrow. To prevent yourself from resembling a werewolf, the secret – which you may only choose to do behind the locked door of a bathroom – is to get hold of a pair of sturdy tweezers and start plucking. Go for about a finger-width gap between your brows. Grab the base of the hair with the tweezers and pull sharply away in the same direction in which the hair grows. You will have a pinprick of pain and may be left with a little temporary redness. If your eyebrows are too bushy, with stray hairs tickling your eyes or forehead, give them the same treatment. Whatever you do, do not shave your eyebrows; the hairs will grow back coarser and blunter, making them more prominent every time they grow back.

Your best weapon against nasal hair is a pair of fine, blunt-ended scissors (or an electric or battery-operated nasal-hair trimmer). Push the end of your nose up to expose your nostrils and trim any protruding hairs. Do not delve deeper than a few millimetres or you may graze the nasal canals. Also, the hairs do provide a worthwhile function in trapping debris and pollution when you breathe in. Never pluck these hairs – apart from making you weep, the exposed follicles could become infected. If you find stray hairs protruding from your ears take the scissors to these, too.

You may wonder what kind of madman would pay good money to have hot wax poured over his back, then have it ripped off, pulling out his body hairs with it. But if you have a hairy back and are sick of being mistaken for a gorilla, it could be your only option.

Waxing is an effective form of hair removal, leaving smooth, hair-free skin for a couple of months before the process needs to be repeated, and is used by professional cyclists and athletes for whom excess body hair can be a hindrance. Check out the beauty pages in your telephone directory to find a suitable salon to have a treatment. Waxing is most commonly associated with women's bodies, so find a venue that is male-friendly – you don't want to find yourself with waxed legs and painted toenails.

Give yourself a hand

All a manicurist will do to your hands (or a pedicurist to your feet) is stuff you can do at home with a couple of tools from a chemist and some decent moisturizing cream. Danielle Winter, a London-based manicurist, starts by cleaning under each nail with a curved metal file before clipping them. She says; 'I would never use scissors, only straight-edged clippers, leaving a thin white strip of nail beyond the finger.' Clippers are far easier to use and control than scissors – most of us can manage to cut the nails on both hands using them. If you get into trouble, keep practising – you can hardly ask your mother after all these years. Turn the back of your hand towards you so you can see your nails clearly and start by clipping the middle of the nail to the required length with small snips before cutting the sides of the nail. Your nails will be easier to cut if you trim them after a bath or shower, which softens both nails and cuticles.

'I file the nails to give a smooth edge using an emery board,' continues Winter. Make sure you work in one direction only across the edge of the nail, which avoids splitting it. 'Then I soak the hands in warm, soapy water for five minutes to soften the skin before pushing back the cuticles with a cuticle stick.' Do not use a hard implement to push back your cuticles, as it could damage your nail growth – you can use the edge of a towel or face cloth to push them back. Cuticles protect nails at their growing point, so do not

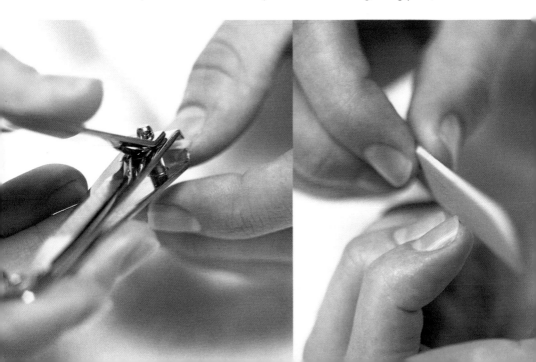

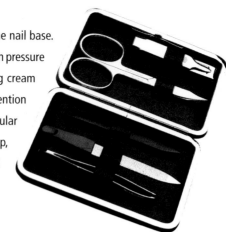

remove them, just keep them in place at the nail base. 'Finally, I massage in hand cream, focusing on pressure points to keep the hands relaxed.' Rubbing cream into your hands is relaxing – pay special attention to the base of each finger and rub in a circular motion. This is the area where calluses develop, and regular use of a rich moisturizing hand cream will stop them in their tracks.

HOME MANICURE

1 Trim your nails with clippers, starting in the centre of the nail and finishing with a couple of snips at the sides.

2 File the edges smooth with a soft emery board, working in one direction only.

3 Soak the hands, then gently push back the cuticles with a cuticle stick.

4 Last of all, massage in some rich, moisturizing hand cream.

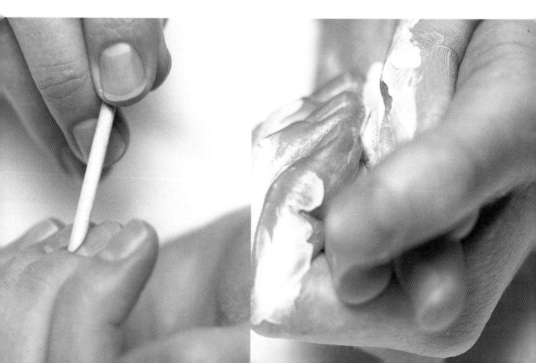

Toeing the line

If it is a struggle to pay attention to your hands, then your feet will hardly get a look-in. Chipped toenails, hard skin and poor cleaning are a recipe for unsightly feet, and though a potential boss will not have a clue what is going on under those smart wing-tip brogues, a hot date could end up calling Environmental Health. They may never be beautiful, but some care and attention make feet feel great and may even cause whoops of delight from your partner, who will no longer turn green every time you remove your socks. If you are lucky, you may even get a foot massage – and a foot massage from the woman in your life is up there with the greatest pleasures known to man (alongside lie-ins and take-out curries – and pretty close to free beer for life).

On an average day feet absorb over 2½ million kg (5½ million lb) of pressure, making them, perhaps, the most hard-working parts of the body while remaining the most neglected. Three implements used regularly will make them feel like star performers that you cannot live without: a pumice stone (a volcanic rock, lightweight and full of holes) or other abrasive skin-removing tool, nail clippers and a moisturizer or foot cream (foot cream should include a natural odour-eater like peppermint). Try to get into the habit of using a pumice stone or a foot file, especially on the edge of your heels where dry, dead skin mostly builds up, every time you bath or shower – the warm water softens the skin, making it easier to remove. Wash your feet daily; it is not good enough just to let the water swish around your feet – use your hands or a cloth to wash your feet and between your toes, then dry them well, too. Follow with a rich moisturizer, which, apart from feeling great while you do it, puts a spring in your step for hours. Good footcare is simple, the only secret is to keep doing it regularly.

HOME PEDICURE

1   After or during your bath or shower, remove any dead skin from your soles and heels by rubbing them gently with a pumice stone or metal foot file.

2   Cut your nails with nail clippers, working from the middle of the nail to the sides and leaving a thin white line at the edge of the nail.

3   Finish off by massaging in a moisturizing foot cream.

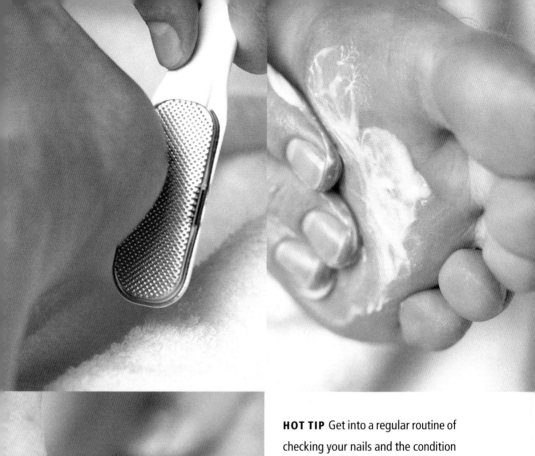

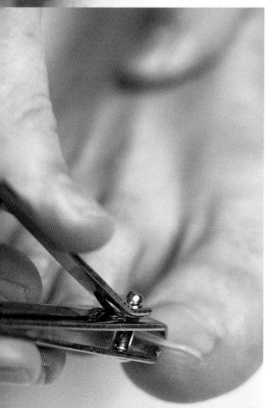

HOT TIP Get into a regular routine of checking your nails and the condition of your feet (about once a week) – you don't want someone else alerting you to jagged toenails ripping through your shoes. And always do your hand and foot regimes in private. For some, as yet unfathomed, reason a man attending to his nails is one of the biggest turn-offs known to women. Careful disposal of nail debris is also advisable; if she steps on one of your toenail clippings you will have more chance of winning a roll-over lottery than ever getting a foot massage.

AVOIDING PROBLEMS

If you wear your shoes too tight your toenails will start growing into your skin, so leave those Hank Wangford winkle-picker cowboy boots at the back of the wardrobe and invest in some well-fitting shoes. Badly trimmed nails can also 'train' the sharp edge of the nail to grow down and into the toe rather than safely over the edge. Ingrown toenails may be an inherited tendency, and are also common in people with wide feet. To make ingrown nails a thing of the past wear shoes with at least 1.5 cm (½ inch) between your big toe and the edge of the shoe, and always cut your toenails straight across – do not trim the corners of your nails or cut them too short, since this can encourage them to grow under the skin. After cutting your toenails run a fingertip over the cut edges to check they feel smooth – a quick rub with an emery board should get rid of any roughness.

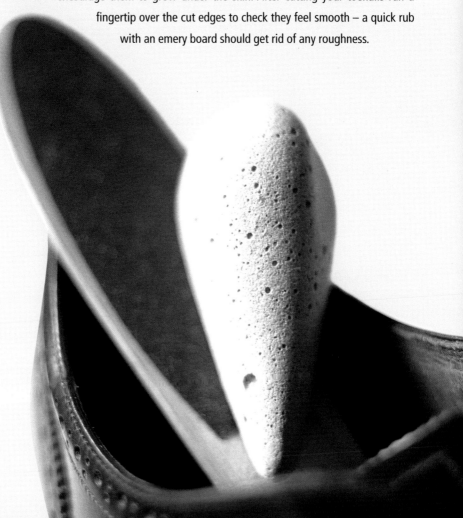

HARVESTING THE CORN

Corns are caused by a build-up of hard, dead skin that forms on the load-bearing parts of your feet to protect the skin, bones and muscles from further wear and tear. If this callus build-up occurs on your toes, and its growth runs rampant, then the dead skin turns into a corn (a deep plug of hard skin that will need to be professionally removed). Visit a reputable pedicurist to have them cut away, or use corn plasters to cure the problem (a circle of felt with a hole in the middle, which takes the pressure off the corn). Similarly, bunions can form on your toes when the friction from tight shoes causes bone to grow in and around the toe joints. If you regularly slough off dry skin and use a moisturizer you should manage to avoid these painful little irritants.

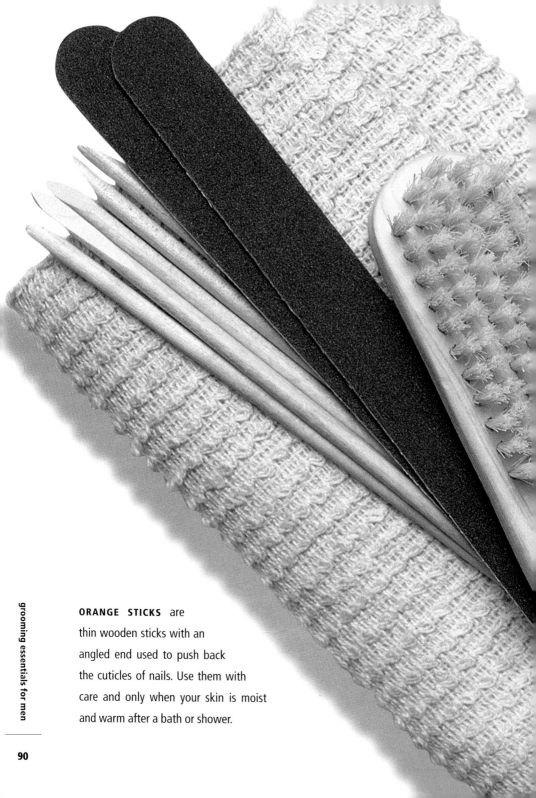

ORANGE STICKS are
thin wooden sticks with an
angled end used to push back
the cuticles of nails. Use them with
care and only when your skin is moist
and warm after a bath or shower.

EMERY BOARDS work like small boards of sandpaper to file down and smooth freshly trimmed nails. To avoid splitting the nail, use an emery board in one direction only across the edge of the nail; this also helps you control how much is removed.

FUNGUS THE BOGEYMAN

It is hard to miss when you are not taking enough care of your feet. You only have to inhale to get more proof than you need. Odour-causing bacteria thrive in warm, moist environments – inside your shoes is their idea of paradise. Wearing leather shoes and pure cotton or wool socks helps in the fight against foot odour, and not wearing trainers (except in the gym) is a good way of avoiding unnecessary sweating. The odour from some trainers could surely be harnessed for biological warfare and used to devastating effect. Use charcoal inserts inside your shoes to kill the aroma and absorb moisture.

If your feet cannot breathe and there is too much moisture and heat around them, it can make you vulnerable to athlete's foot, an irritating fungal infection that is usually picked up in gym or pool changing rooms, or wherever people walk around with bare feet – even naturists wear sandals. You have probably got it if your feet burn, itch and look dry or scaly – especially between your toes. Over-the-counter remedies are a starting point and always wearing rubber shoes in public showers helps avoid contracting it or passing it on. If the problem persists seek medical advice.

Oral lessons

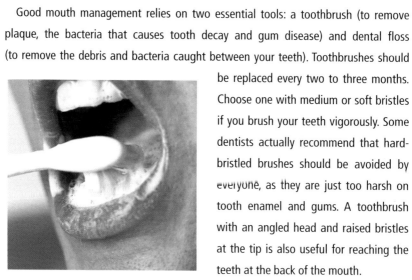

Your skin may now be looking better than ever – clean, smooth and blemish-free, but open your mouth and those greying tombstone pegs are going to let you down – and as if anyone could ignore that rich aroma pouring from your mouth, too. Oral hygiene and good teeth management are as much a health issue as a grooming one. As Dr Alfred Agbenyega, a London-based dentist remarks, 'To have good-looking teeth and healthy gums not only makes you look younger, it also proves that you are looking after your mouth properly.' And if your teeth are not clean, people will start to wonder about all your other hygiene habits. Furthermore, what woman with reasonable eyesight and a functioning sense of smell is going to voluntarily put her mouth anywhere near yours without a high standard of mouth hygiene on your part?

Good mouth management relies on two essential tools: a toothbrush (to remove plaque, the bacteria that causes tooth decay and gum disease) and dental floss (to remove the debris and bacteria caught between your teeth). Toothbrushes should

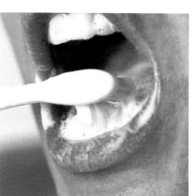

be replaced every two to three months. Choose one with medium or soft bristles if you brush your teeth vigorously. Some dentists actually recommend that hard-bristled brushes should be avoided by everyone, as they are just too harsh on tooth enamel and gums. A toothbrush with an angled head and raised bristles at the tip is also useful for reaching the teeth at the back of the mouth.

DR ALFRED AGBENYEGA'S THREE TIPS FOR GOOD BRUSHING

1   To prevent excessive wear of the tooth enamel and recession of the gums, use a brush that has soft or medium bristles, and replace it at least every three months.

2   Brushing up and down or across the teeth is equally effective at removing plaque from between the junction of the gum and teeth.

3   Brush your teeth twice a day for at least two minutes each time.

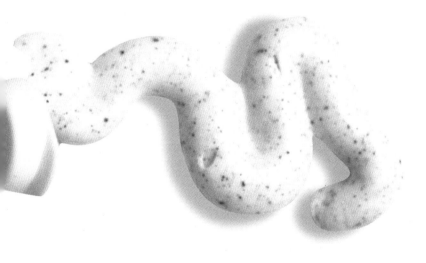

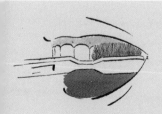 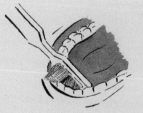 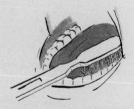

Clean your teeth twice a day, taking care to reach the teeth at the back of your mouth and making sure you brush the outer and inner surfaces, as well as the biting part.

FLOSSING

Dental floss is not just for people who are hygiene fixated – we should all be doing it at the end of every day. Otherwise that speck of chicken from last week's roast, which brushing alone will not remove, will quietly nurture a host of tooth-boring bacteria and may cause a gum infection as well as a cavity.

To remove bacteria from in between your teeth, take a 30-cm (1-foot) strand of floss (waxed versions are gentler on your gums – and you can even buy mint-flavoured floss), wrap the ends around your index fingers leaving about 10 cm (4 inches) to do the work. Start with the floss against the gum between a pair of teeth and gently draw it straight out away from the gum, taking any food debris with it; repeat if necessary. Take care not to bring the floss down too heavily onto your gums, as it can make them bleed.

NO MORE NASTY NIFFS

Almost more worrying than the state of our teeth, suffering from bad breath is one of our most cherished fears. This is hardly surprising if our staple diet is a combination of beer, vindaloo curry and garlic bread. Yet even the smell from these pongy foods can be easily overcome – chewing raw parsley is a good odour neutralizer – and our fear of bad breath nearly always far outweighs the reality. Bad breath is caused by bacteria at the back of the tongue and sides of the mouth, which a toothbrush is unable to reach. However, it will help if you gently rub your brush over your tongue when you clean your teeth. Regularly scraping the back of the tongue with an inverted teaspoon or special scraper is also a good idea if you fear bad breath. You will probably not

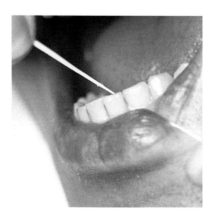

know that you have smelly breath unless an honest friend tells you. 'Your own sense of smell can't detect your own bad breath,' says Dr Richter of the USA's first bad-breath centre in Philadelphia (the Richter Center). 'And it won't help to breathe into your cupped palms or lick the back of your hand,' he explains, 'as your breath can take on an odour simply by mixing with air.'

A mouthwash will not necessarily solve the problem. According to Richter, it is probably just masking one smell with another more pleasant one, usually mint. It is far better to scrape your tongue, brush your teeth twice a day and regularly floss between your teeth. If the problem persists see your dentist.

VIRTUAL WHITENESS

Hydrogen peroxide is the wonder chemical used in both professional and home teeth-bleaching kits. According to Dr Agbenyega, 'Bleaching gives a more youthful smile by lightening your teeth, which can massively boost your self-confidence.' Bleaching can be done at home with a kit or professionally by a dentist, in which case peroxide is painted onto the teeth and the chemical reaction is enhanced by shining an ultraviolet light onto them. Home bleaching kits (which have weaker chemicals than those used by professionals but are still effective) contain a tray in which you immerse your teeth, usually for a few hours every day for up to a week (follow the instructions carefully). The down side to bleaching is that it can cause temporary sensitivity and discomfort, and should be avoided by people whose teeth have particular sensitivity to hot and cold.

DR ALFRED AGBENYEGA'S SIX TIPS FOR HEALTHY TEETH AND GUMS

1   Avoid hard-headed brushes as they can cause long-term damage to both teeth and gums.

2   If you have run out of toothpaste, use your toothbrush anyway as it is the action of the bristles against the teeth and gums that removes plaque.

3   Do use toothpaste, though, since it contains both antibacterial agents and fluoride, which protects enamel from decay, and leaves the mouth fresh.

4   There are many ways of brushing your teeth but the key points are: do not use excessive pressure, which will leave your gums sore; replace your brush every two to three months (a worn-out brush is useless); do not brush your teeth more than twice a day, as this can cause receding gums and enamel wear.

5   Avoid sugary snacks, as sugar in the mouth attracts bacteria whose by-product is acid, which weakens the tooth enamel and leads to decay.

6   Have a check-up every six months.

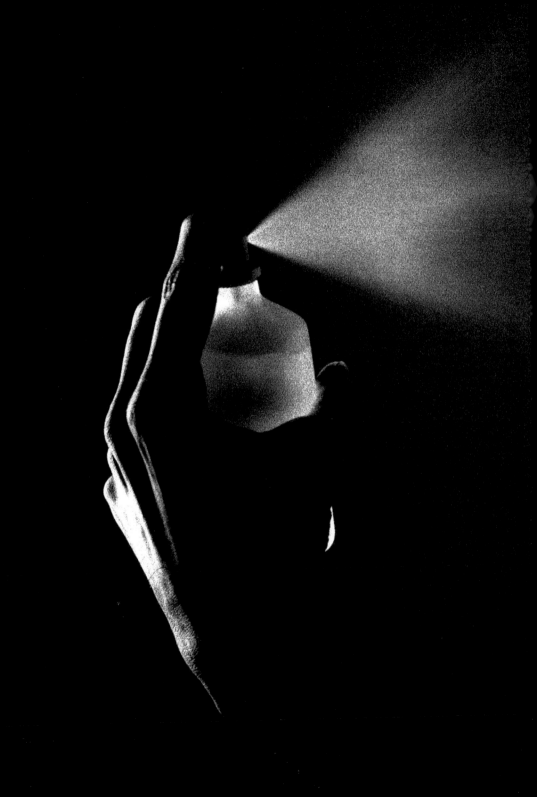

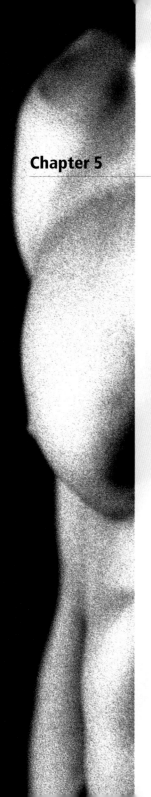

Chapter 5

fragrance

THE FRAGRANCE YOU WEAR GIVES A
PERSONAL MESSAGE TO THE WORLD
ABOUT HOW YOU SEE YOURSELF AND
HOW YOU WANT TO BE REGARDED, SO
IT IS WORTH INVESTIGATING THE
VARIOUS TYPES AND FAMILIES OF SCENT
ON THE MARKET. YOU MAY BE WEARING
CARGO PANTS AND A T-SHIRT, BUT SPLASH
ON SOME SOPHISTICATED FRENCH PONG
AND TO ALL WOMANKIND YOU ARE A
DEAD RINGER FOR SACHA DISTEL.

MANY MEN CHOOSE NOT TO WEAR ANY
KIND OF FRAGRANCE AT ALL, BUT IF YOU
DO AND YOU GO RUNNING OR TO THE
GYM EVERY DAY, REAPPLYING YOUR
FRAGRANCE AFTER A BATH OR SHOWER
WILL BECOME A BORE. CONVENIENTLY,
MANY FRAGRANCE RANGES NOW
INCLUDE BODY LOTIONS, SHOWER GELS,
SOAPS AND DEODORANTS, WHICH ARE
AN EASY WAY OF APPLYING SCENT
WHILE CARRYING OUT YOUR USUAL
GROOMING ROUTINE.

message in a bottle

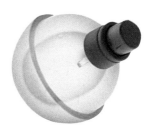

IT MAY SEEM STARTLINGLY OBVIOUS, BUT OUR **SENSE OF SMELL** is our most underestimated sense, yet if you smell good you are likely to gain a more positive reaction from people. We talk about love at first sight, but we should really talk about love at first sniff, according to Alan Hirsch, a neurologist and psychiatrist with the Smell and Taste Treatment and Research Foundation in Chicago. He explains, 'Odours from the environment and other people cause us to have an emotional reaction, and then we make a cognitive decision to rationalize our feelings.' In other words, we give a positive association to people and things that smell good and a negative one to those that smell unpleasant. Try splashing on Eau de Pig Farm if you have any doubt about this assertion.

The words 'scent of a man' probably make you think of those nasty whiffs in changing rooms, but it need not be so. In the world's fragrance industry barely a month goes by without the launch of an exciting new aroma to tickle the olfactory senses of men, who are encouraged to wear it, and women, who are encouraged to be lured by it (that's the idea, anyhow). So with a little trial and error, you should be able to find a fragrance that matches your requirements.

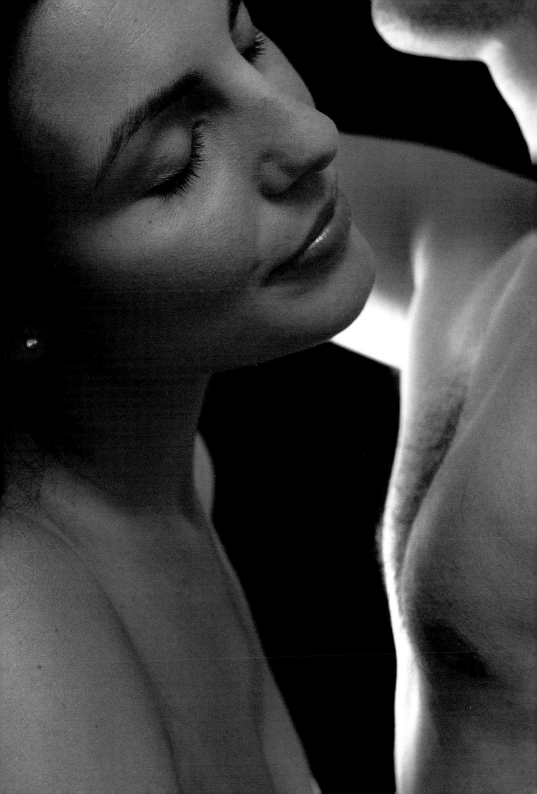

Shopping for smell

Facing a men's fragrance counter for the first time can be a confusing experience – there are so many smells to choose from and the pitch from the sales person is likely to be a hard sell without your best interests at heart – after all, their agenda is to shift as many bottles of scent as possible and not necessarily work out every individual's needs. You do not want to walk away with a bottle of liquid testosterone or smelling like a lavender bush, but with a bit of prior preparation and an idea of the kind of fragrance you are looking for, when you want to wear it and for what purpose (smelling good is a fair goal) you should not end up with an expensive mistake.

It is a necessary cliché, so it has to be stated: the same aroma can smell different depending on who is wearing it, so test any potential fragrance on your own skin before purchasing it – the wrist is ideal (if you run out of wrists a sample can be sprayed onto a card, but this will not tell you what the fragrance smells like on you). Young women have the strongest sense of smell, so take one with you when you go shopping.

There are three categories of men's fragrance – cologne, eau de cologne and aftershave, with cologne having the highest concentration of pure fragrance (usually a blend of essential oils or a chemical imitation of a naturally occurring aroma), while aftershave has the least.

COLOGNE is the strongest fragrance a man can buy, but should not be confused with women's perfume, which is an even more concentrated form of scent. Cologne should be used sparingly because of its strength and, although it is expensive, it is potentially the most economic because a little can last up to six hours.

EAU DE COLOGNE is a weaker form of cologne, which can be splashed liberally on your body, neck and even hair – an increasingly popular way for men to wear fragrance – and the scent will last for approximately four hours.

AFTERSHAVE is the weakest aroma but it can pack quite a stinging punch since it has the highest alcohol content. The alcohol acts as an astringent on your beard area and as an antiseptic to clean and protect freshly shaved skin. However, alcohol is also very drying, so avoid putting aftershave on your face unless you have very oily skin.

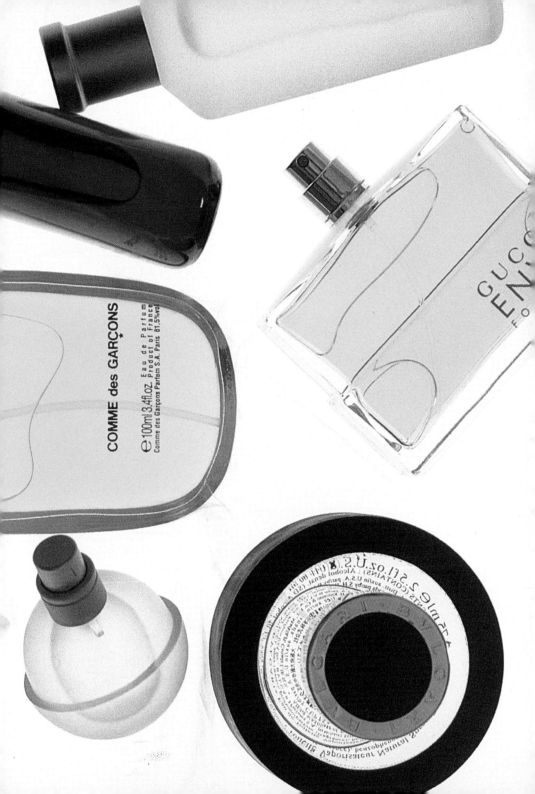

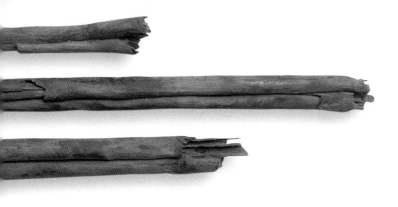

Take notes

Classic fragrances have three layers of scent, known as notes – top, middle and base. The top note is the first smell you pick up immediately after applying a scent and it only lasts for about 15 minutes before fading. This initial hit then progresses to the middle note, the main core of the scent, which should last for another hour or so. Since this is the heart of the aroma, this should be the moment when you decide if the fragrance really suits you or not. When buying scent try waiting for as long as possible in the store before making your purchase to see whether you like this layer of the scent on you or not. The middle note then becomes the base note after you have been wearing the fragrance for a while and it has mingled with your personal odour and the individual chemistry of your skin. The base or bottom note is the final signature of the fragrance and can linger for many hours after applying the product. Because scent blends with your own body odour, heat and sweat from your body will emphasize the aroma – so never wear a cologne when you are going to the gym. In normal conditions, fragrance can last up to four hours, depending on how oily or dry your skin is (oily skin holds fragrance for longer).

It is also true that the same fragrance can smell differently on you depending on what you have eaten and what soaps you have used, and even what time of year it is. Lighter citrus fragrances with a pineapple or citrus top note, or fragrances with marine notes, are best for the daytime and summer, for instance, while scents that are more woody and spicy work well for special occasions and in the evening and winter months. Keeping two or three favourite fragrances at one time to use according to your mood and the occasion is a good idea.

Essential stuff

Essential oils are highly concentrated extracts of flowers, plants and herbs, which, apart from usually smelling pretty good, can be used to enhance your mood, alleviate stress, cure headaches and aid digestion. Here are five essences to keep in your bathroom cabinet; add a few drops to your bath whenever you feel under the weather (these oils are so concentrated that one or two drops are all you need to use at a time).

LAVENDER is the one to go for if you are only going to use one oil. A couple of drops on your pillow will aid relaxation and sleep; used in your bath it can help depression and applied in a cold compress it helps ease swelling and bruising.

PEPPERMINT is a decongestant that will help clear nasal blockages. Add a couple of drops to a bowl of hot water, place a towel over your head and inhale the vapours for instant relief. This can help cure headaches, too.

TEA TREE is a powerful antiviral, antibacterial oil that can be used directly on the skin to clear up spots and rashes, and helps cure warts, herpes and athlete's foot.

EUCALYPTUS is antiseptic, so add it to your bath water when you have a cold or flu to help relieve a sore throat, congestion and sinusitis.

ROSEMARY stimulates both the memory and mental faculties. A few drops in your bath after a workout will relax strained muscles; and it can also cure dandruff – rub a few drops into your hair after washing while your hair is still wet.

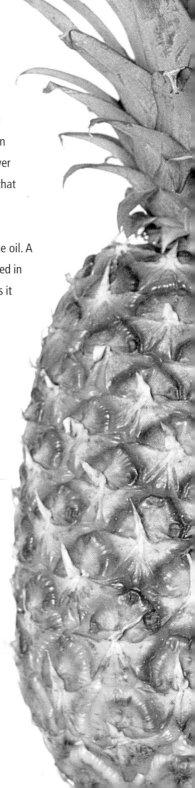

ORIENTAL

warm, sensual, seductive, mysterious

JOOP! Homme, JOOP!
Obsession for Men, Calvin Klein
Le Male, Jean Paul Gaultier
Habit Rouge, Guerlain

WOODY

warm, elegant, precious, mysterious

Polo, Ralph Lauren
Gucci Envy for Men, Gucci
Fahrenheit, Christian Dior
Héritage, Guerlain

SPICY

fiery, exotic, rugged, expressive

Égoïste, Chanel
Armani eau pour Homme, Giorgio Armani
Xeryus Rouge, Guerlain
Santos, Cartier

CITRUS

vital, fresh, natural, invigorating

Acqua di Giò pour Homme, Giorgio Armani
Eau Sauvage, Christian Dior
L'eau d'Issey pour Homme, Issey Miyake
Rochas Man, Rochas

Fragrance families

The four bands of fragrance families in the chart on the left indicate broadly the individual characteristics of some of the top men's scents, describing them as oriental, woody, spicy or citrus. But in addition to being categorized into one of the fragrance families, there is also more specific and detailed information that you can only gain by trying out the scent on your own body and seeing how it combines with your natural odour.

Acqua di Giò pour Homme by Giorgio Armani, for instance, belongs to the citrus family. In addition to its fruity characteristics, which give it freshness, it also has a marine note, making it smell sporty and summery. A world away from the Armani scent is Gucci Envy for Men, which is a woody fragrance that also has amber and oriental notes.

When you are trying out a new scent, the two most important deciding factors are: do you like the smell on your own skin – immediately after applying it and a while later – and does anyone back away from you gagging? Get those two criteria right and, as well as making you feel good, your smell cannot fail to enhance your image, completing another small, but necessary, step to becoming irresistible to women.

Keep it simple

If you use a fragranced soap when you wash in the morning, followed by a perfumed deodorant and then a splash of cologne, you will be a walking cocktail of different aromas. If you do want to wear cologne, it is far better to use fragrance-free products on your body, or at least use products from the same range (although you may find the scent becomes overpowering).

Apply fragrance only after washing yourself – never use it to cover up a less-than-clean body; it doesn't work and you will end up smelling of a sickly combination of body odour and musky sandalwood. Also, do not apply too much cologne. Obviously this is a relative rule, but less is usually very definitely more in the fragrance game (your smart, expensive product will last longer, too). A few minutes after applying cologne, it becomes invisible to our own nose, but that doesn't mean it is not capable of knocking over others at 60 paces. 'You want your fragrance to be wonderful and diffusive, not to invade the space of others. Only someone very close to you should notice your smell. It should not hang in the air around you,' according to Natalie Hinden-Kuhles, vice-president of fragrance development at Revlon.

Where to splash it

Wearing fragrance where you would like to be kissed – Coco Chanel's famous maxim to women – does not really translate too well for men. Far better to keep to familiar territory, such as behind your ears, your neck and upper chest, and even your hair (apply some cologne to your hands first and then rub it through your locks). Most fragrances, even some aftershaves, are too harsh to put on your face and the alcohol found in most of them is too drying. Keep a bottle of fragrance with you if you go out straight after work and have a quick refreshing splash in the gents before hitting the night (a fresh-smelling fragrance can give your spirits a boost, too).

Cooling off

If you do splash out big money on your fragrance, keep it in a cool, dark place – even the fridge – where it will last longer and stay fresher, and never leave a bottle of cologne in direct sunlight, which will ruin the smell and colour. Air will also affect the fragrance and colour, so always replace the lid after use.

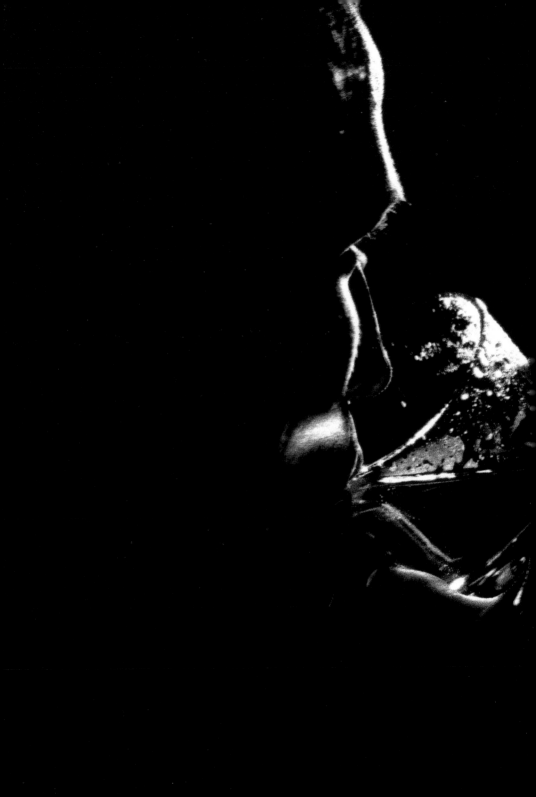

fashion & style

YOUR SKIN MIGHT BE SMOOTH, YOUR SHAVING ROUTINE EXEMPLARY AND YOUR HAIRCUT FEATURED IN THE WINDOW OF YOUR LOCAL BARBER SHOP, BUT YOUR CLOTHES COULD BE MAKING YOU LOOK LIKE SOMEONE WHO HAS PICKED UP THE WRONG LAUNDRY. YOU NEED TO LEARN A FEW CLOTHING BASICS TO BE CONSIDERED A TRULY WELL-GROOMED MAN.

UNLIKE WOMEN, WHO HAVE TO PICK THEIR WAY THROUGH THE FICKLE WORLD OF FLUCTUATING HEMLINES AND CONSTANTLY EVOLVING COLOURS PRODUCED BY A GALAXY OF BRANDS, MEN REALLY HAVE NO EXCUSE FOR GETTING IT WRONG. MEN'S CLOTHING HAS BEEN BASED UPON TROUSERS, SHIRTS AND JACKETS FOR THE WHOLE OF THE TWENTIETH CENTURY. WHILE OUR CASUAL GEAR, A CLASSIC JEANS AND T-SHIRT COMBINATION, HAS NEVER LOOKED OUT OF FASHION.

step into style

WOMEN'S FASHION MAY BE PARTICULARLY FICKLE, BUT **MENSWEAR**
evolves much more slowly and there is little sign that certain kinds of clothes
are suddenly going to look old-fashioned and unstylish. Classic chinos with a
white T-shirt and a V-neck sweater is a hard look to get wrong. While a classic
three-button, single-breasted suit (with flat-front trousers and a narrow leg)
is another wardrobe staple that provides a huge variety of looks depending
on what you decide to wear with it. For instance, a simple V-neck T-shirt for a
casual take or a pale blue shirt worn with a silk tie, which will stand you in
good stead for interviews, impressing your parents-in-law and courts of law
(well, you never know).

So, as a man, there is little excuse for not dressing well – although try telling
that to the myriad of unstylish men that we pass every day, who sport such
arrestable offences as a nylon lilac shirt under a grey leather 1970s-style
blouson. And get over any prejudice you may have that dressing well requires
you to sell the family silver – it doesn't. What it does require is simply a little
thought to work out what you need to wear and for what occasion. Then follow
a few basic rules about what goes with what and how to recognize the best
styles and cuts to suit your body shape. (For example, if you are built like Danny
de Vito, never be seen in a broad-shouldered double-breasted suit in a window-
pane check – you will look like someone who has been steamrollered.)

Suits you, sir

Dressing well is not about buying the latest designer jacket, wearing it and imagining everyone is thinking, 'What a cool, stylish guy.' Rather, you should be dressing to suit your body shape and the kind of world in which you have to work and function. Having to wear a suit to work can feel boring and conventional, but a huge benefit is that the process of getting dressed every morning is relatively hassle free (apart from when that half-Windsor knot just will not sit properly). And if you do have to wear a suit, the colour, weight of cloth and cut will all play a key role in how it looks on you. If it is acceptable to wear casual clothes to work instead of a suit, getting dressed can still be a minefield: should chinos regarded as being as casual as jeans, for instance? Usually not. However, even more fraught with danger is the question of what to wear in the evening, at the weekend and on an important date, and this is where most of us slip up or at least get nervous. Ditch the appliquéd-teddy-bear jumper your mum gave you in 1989, anything in fuschia pink and clothes that do not fit you any more (and are unlikely to again). Make a trip to your local charity shop with anything you have not worn in the last year and are pretty sure you will not wear again. These items just take up space and crease the other clothes on the rail for the next year, too – and you never know, you just might pick up a bargain original Pierre Cardin coat while you are in there. Also, use women as style gurus – few are the women without strong opinions about what men should or should not wear, so team up with a stylish female friend when you go shopping and see what she thinks suits you.

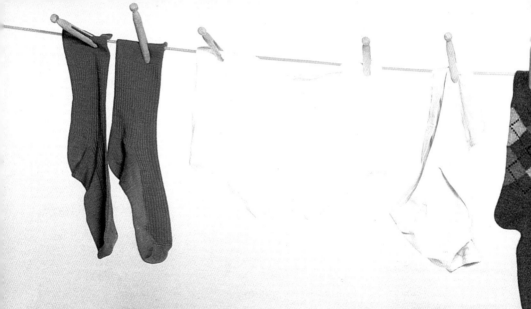

To make the most of your clothes, stick to basic colours that suit you. Many men with pale, northern-European colouring look ill wearing black, which is just too dark; far better, then, to stick to navy, which is as smart as black but more flattering. If you have a navy Mac, navy trousers (or dark jeans) and a contrasting beige sweater worn over a white T-shirt, you will look stylish without looking overly casual. The colour of your eyes is a good indication of the kinds of colours to go for. Shades of blue suit those with blue eyes, and so on. It does not have to be an exact match, just closely related.

The most important rule of good dressing is to keep it simple. When it comes to clothes, leave trickiness and flamboyance to rock stars and entertainers. Those black leather biker-style trousers may look great on the back of a Harley but they look ludicrous in a bar or supermarket. Err on the side of caution in both colour and cut and make an individual statement through accessories and details. It may only be a pale blue V-neck sweater, but if it is made of cashmere it will be fantastically soft, warm and lightweight. Choose a cashmere and wool mix for overcoats and jackets – the extra expense will be more than compensated for by the feel of luxury. Menswear is less about ostentation and more about subtlety.

Whatever you wear, wear it with confidence. If you have got on a new shirt and tie combo that is a bit more colourful that you are used to you will only draw attention to it by feeling self-conscious. Far better to behave as if you have always worn such gear, making people more likely to think it looks great.

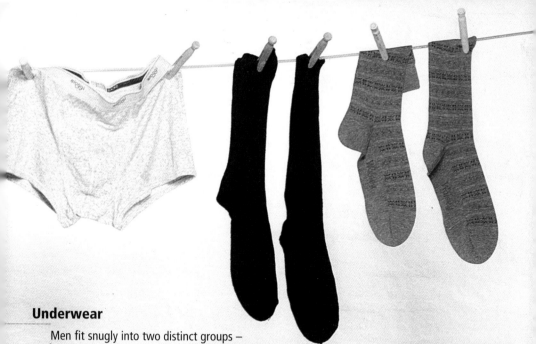

Underwear

Men fit snugly into two distinct groups –

those who wear briefs and those who wear boxers – rare is the man who will sport both (especially at the same time); some even go combat style with no underwear at all (but this could weigh heavily on your laundry bill). Whatever your preference, for sport wear supportive Lycra and cotton mix briefs, which will keep things under control better than loose shorts. Avoid novelty underwear at all times; you never know when trouser removal will be required and those 'kiss me quick' briefs could leave you squirming.

Belt up

Simple rules to wearing the right belt:

- Wear the same colour belt as your shoes.
- Avoid big buckles that draw attention to your waist and any excess poundage you could be carrying there.
- Lighter-coloured and fabric belts should only be worn with casual clothes.
- Make sure that when you wear a dark suit your belt is darker than the fabric (which usually means black).
- If you can afford it go for best-quality full-grain leather, or a cheaper belt that has been treated to make it look grainy.

The right suit

A LEAN MAN has long limbs and should counteract his vertical height by wearing clothes that give him the appearance of bulk. Double-breasted styles with plaid patterns will give the illusion of greater girth. A window-pane check (large squares) can be subtle but still imply bulk. A bold Prince of Wales check would work well, too. Lean men should avoid vertical lines, such as pinstripes, which will only emphasize their narrowness.

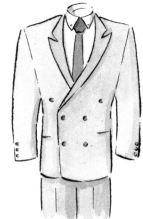

A NORMAL OR REGULAR BODY SHAPE, which is neither lean nor stocky, with the body's components roughly in proportion with each other, is the most versatile to clothe, as you can get away with almost any style. Choose more fashionable cuts of suit, which tend to be on the leaner side these days. Flat-front trousers and single-breasted contoured jackets (cut to the body) will all look good on you. Either patterned suits or plain can be worn and look equally good.

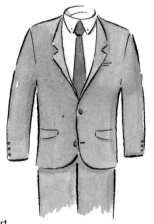

A STOCKY BODY is characterized by a thick neck, short limbs and a square, sturdy torso (think Danny De Vito but with a bit more height). With this body shape you are trying to create the illusion of tallness to counteract the squareness of your body. Vertical lines, such as pin- or chalk-stripes, and a high-buttoned jacket (of at least three or even four buttons) finishing just below the chest will take the eye away from any thickness around your waist. Avoid turn-ups or cuffs at the bottom of the trousers, which foreshorten the leg, and avoid checks and plaids, which will only emphasize the width of your shape rather than counteract it.

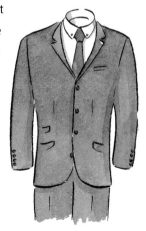

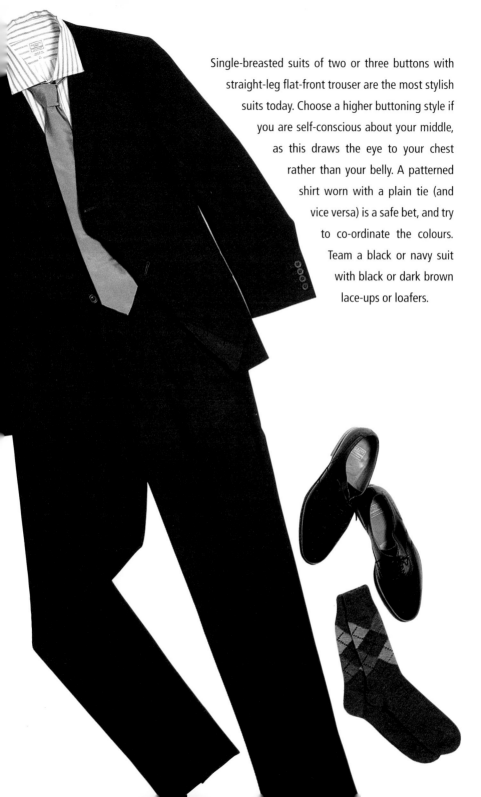

Single-breasted suits of two or three buttons with straight-leg flat-front trouser are the most stylish suits today. Choose a higher buttoning style if you are self-conscious about your middle, as this draws the eye to your chest rather than your belly. A patterned shirt worn with a plain tie (and vice versa) is a safe bet, and try to co-ordinate the colours. Team a black or navy suit with black or dark brown lace-ups or loafers.

THE SHIRT AND TIE

There is a limit to how much individuality you can show with a navy suit until you add your shirt and tie. This is one of the few areas of smart dress where you can really express yourself. A word of warning, however, go down the novelty tie route at your peril – that Tweetie Pie motif will not make women think you are cute and nor will your boss regard you as suitably mature for the corporate fast track.

The classic navy suit combined with a white shirt can be worn with a tie of almost any colour or pattern, but one of plain navy will look smartest. Sheer silks in plain colours can look smart, too. For a change, experiment with texture rather than patterns and wear a knitted or woven tie. If you want to wear a patterned tie be sure that your shirt is plain and vice versa. Never feel obliged to wear a tie just because it was a present.

As with the suit itself, go for the best quality shirts and ties that you can afford. Silk ties are infinitely nicer and hang better than ones of man-made fibres, while shirts made from 100 per cent cotton look smarter, are more comfortable to wear and let your skin breathe. Bespoke shirts are a good idea if you have particularly long arms or a very thick neck as they are made expressly to fit your body. Collars should always be of a classic style, without buttons (cut-away if you like to wear a big knot), and double cuffs that require cufflinks tend to look smarter than single-layer button-up cuffs.

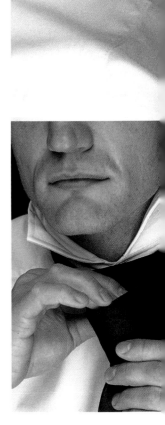

HALF-WINDSOR KNOT

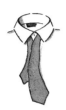   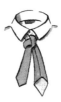 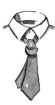

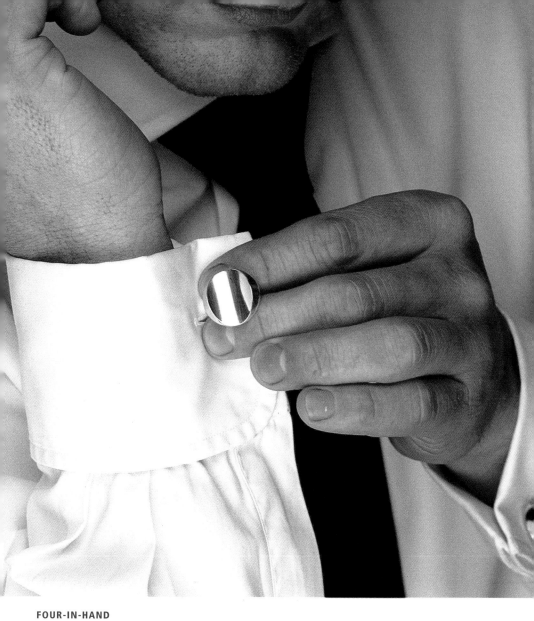

FOUR-IN-HAND

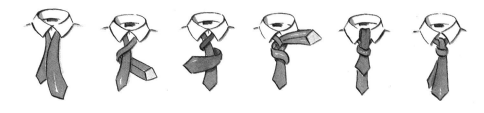

The casual basics

The classic items that are found in almost every man's wardrobe have been around for years and are ageless. You really cannot go wrong with a regular cut of jeans, sturdy dark brown boots, a casual jacket, a white T-shirt and V-neck sweater in a plain knit. All wardrobes should contain these items and variations of them, along with your suit and a selection of shirts and ties, a coat and a raincoat.

Of course, it is fine to recommend these clothing basics but walk into any jeans store and you will be faced with an alarming number of racks of different styles, cuts and colours of denim (see pages 118–19). Keep things simple by ignoring what the sales assistants say – they will point you towards those lose-cut hipsters worn by hip-hop stars that have more yards of fabric than schooner mainsail. Rather, choose a classic five-pocket straight-leg style (this cut has been around for the best part of 100 years so it must be doing something for those who wear it).

THE WRONG TROUSERS

Although fit is the key factor in wearing the right trousers, the cut can flatter or undermine your best intentions. Here are some guidelines to help you make sure you get the most from your strides.

- Apart from jeans and some very casual styles of trousers you should always wear your trousers on your waist (not below it). Every man – even the slimmest – has a slight bulge below the waist, so if your waistband is on your waist this bulge is disguised. Wear your trousers below the bulge, however, and you are merely emphasizing your girth.
- If your trousers do not reach your waist, the rise is too short (the distance between the crotch and the waistband). Choose styles with a deeper rise so that they comfortably reach your waist.
- Wear your trousers long enough so that a break forms in the crease on the top of your shoes, and the fabric should rest about 2.5 cm (1 inch) above the heel at the back.
- Straight-leg trousers are the most flattering shape and flat-front styles (no pleats) are the more current look. Stockier bodies may need one or two pleats, which create extra fabric to accommodate a larger rear end.

GET YOURSELF SOME KHAKIS

Chinos, combats, khakis are all pretty much the same thing and describe cotton canvas trousers (most often in beige), which are smarter than jeans but just as comfortable and relaxed to wear. 'They are the ultimate casual alternative to jeans,' says Mark Alden Lukas of the American design house Perry Ellis. 'Slightly dressier but not a pair of dress trousers. The colour is a classic neutral – it goes with so much; and the fabric is so durable.'

The name khaki is derived from the Persian word, *khak*, meaning dust or dirt, and the trousers date back to 19th-century army camouflage (the original colour was created by dyeing white cotton with tea). With versions that have flat fronts or pleats at the waist, and pockets on the leg (combat trousers) or just a single pocket at the back (chinos), there is a style of khaki's to suit everyone.

You can dress up your classic chinos with a shirt and blazer, although they look best of all with relaxed knitwear (sweaters to you) and button-down collar shirts. Combat trousers, loose-fitting or slim-leg, are the more streetwise alternative – the staple uniform of most people below the age of 35. These now come in many other fabrics than the traditional cotton canvas, including linen, moleskin, nylon and even parachute silk. The more casual style of combat pants are best worn with trainers, T-shirts, fleeces and body-warmers for urban cool.

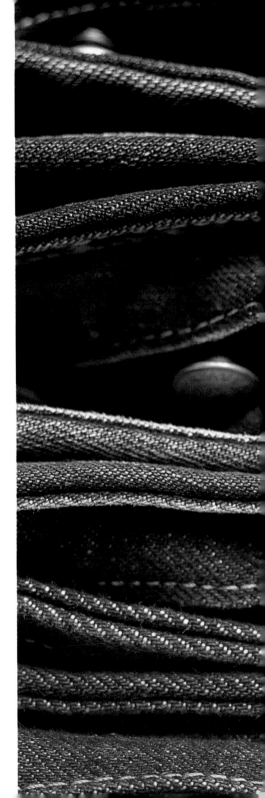

GET THE RIGHT JEANS

Step into any jeans store and you are presented with a mind-boggling selection of styles, colours, button or zip fastenings, weights and finishes. Here is some of the terminology explained to take the fear out of jeans shopping (after all, we all own at least one pair according to statistics).

REGULAR FIT This classic style is cut to the contour of your body. The straight-leg version is about 40 cm (16 inches) wide at the ankles.

RELAXED OR EASY FIT These should provide another centimetre (½ inch) in the seat, thigh, leg and knee, and taper to a 38-cm (15-inch) width at the ankle. This style is a better choice for men with a stockier build.

LOOSE OR BAGGY FIT OR WIDE-LEG This is very young, hip-hop style, usually worn low-slung with some branded underwear peaking over the top. Only wear these if you are under 22 years old and have got a don't-mess-with-me attitude.

STRAIGHT CUT This means that the trouser leg has the same width all the way down the leg; it is generally a tight cut and looks good only on slim men.

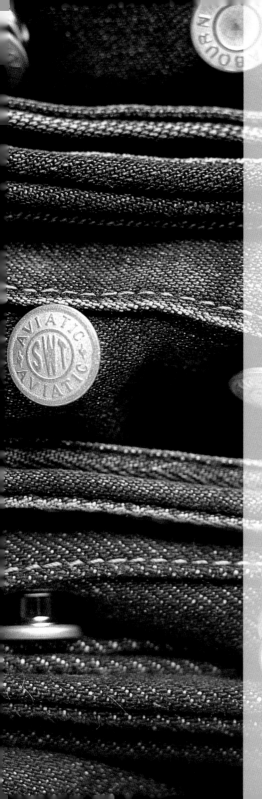

BOOT CUT This is a traditional cowboy style that is cut a bit wider at the ankle to accommodate boots, and consequently looks best when you are wearing some.

FLARES These add about 2.5 cm (1 inch) to the trouser leg, beginning just below the knee. Flares disappeared with the dinosaurs, but some fashion magazines would still have us wear them. Not for the faint-hearted.

BEST FOOT FORWARD

Those smart wing-tip brogues that get admiring glances from you boss are hardly going to look right with your jeans or chinos. If you do not feel comfortable in trainers, why not choose casual loafers in tan or beige suede, which look great with jeans and a chunky matching belt? Most boots, from biker styles to lace-ups, look good with jeans – just don't tuck them in.

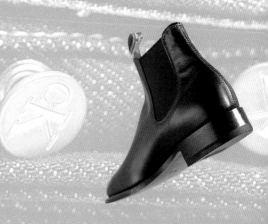

Black tie

Chances are, if you work in the corporate world, your partner is running the country or you enjoy mimicking a penguin, you will be called upon to wear black tie from time to time. This occasion should never be taken as an opportunity to try to compete with your partner and see how much flamboyance you can get away with, since the whole etiquette of black tie is that men dress soberly in a formal uniform to complement the sartorial extravagance and theatricality of the women at the theatre, party or fund-raising event.

Choose to buy or hire a suit in either midnight navy (the darkest shade of navy) or in classic black. If you have a broader body, remember that a single-breasted version will be more slimming than a double-breasted style. A white dress shirt with a bow tie are the only essential gear you can wear it with. Without question, do not even entertain thoughts of wearing a dark T-shirt or an ordinary open-neck shirt (however smart), or elaborate studs or a regular black tie instead of a classic dicky bow – you will not only embarrass yourself but your partner, too. Cummerbunds are, of course, acceptable, but they rarely look good, making you resemble a second-rate wine waiter rather than a suave smoothie. It is also

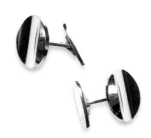

fine to wear a handkerchief in your breast pocket, but only a white one really looks smart. Fold it twice to form a double triangle, turn in two of the points so they meet in the centre, insert it into the pocket and fan out the point. Flamboyant waistcoats with gold buttons, top hats and capes, silver-topped canes and other paraphernalia are just too old-fashioned for today's events, unless, of course, you are rather eccentric and are happy to look like you have just wandered off the set of a period drama. Knotting a bow tie correctly takes a bit of patience and practice (see below), but if it gets the better of you it is fine to wear an elasticated ready-tied version (in fact, it is hard to tell the difference). Bow ties come in many fabrics, colours and patterns, but it is usually advisable not to express your exuberant personality through that route and, especially on more formal occasions, stick to wearing a traditional black tie. Also, wear highly polished or patent shoes with black tie.

BOW TIE

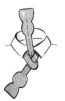

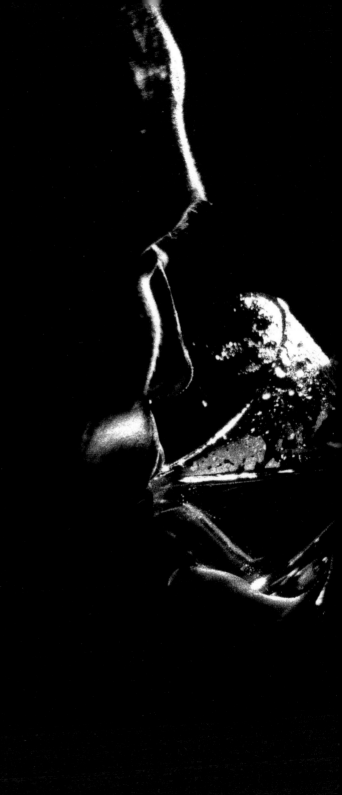

Chapter 7

healthy living

TAKING REGULAR EXERCISE, KEEPING STRESS LEVELS UNDER CONTROL, GETTING ENOUGH RESTORATIVE SLEEP AND EATING NUTRITIOUS FOOD WILL BE OF MORE BENEFIT TO YOUR LOOKS – NOT TO MENTION YOUR HEALTH – THAN ANYTHING YOU SLAP ON YOUR SKIN. IT IS ALL VERY WELL HAVING A BATHROOM CABINET FULL OF EXPENSIVE CREAMS AND POTIONS, BUT IF YOU ARE CONSTANTLY BURNING THE CANDLE AT BOTH ENDS YOU WILL END UP LOOKING A MESS BEFORE YOU CAN SAY, 'LINE THEM UP BARMAN'.

THESE FOUR AREAS WILL TAKE YOU WELL BEYOND THE OBVIOUS CONCERNS OF GROOMING AND, IN COMBINATION WITH EACH OTHER, CAN IMPROVE THE QUALITY OF YOUR LIFE, HEALTH AND ABILITY TO WARD OFF DISEASE. LOOK AFTER YOURSELF ON THE INSIDE AS WELL AS THE OUTSIDE AND YOU WILL LIVE AND LOOK YOUNGER FOR LONGER.

grooming on the inside

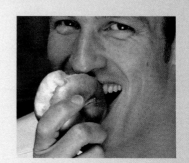

DOING THE RIGHT THING IN **THE BATHROOM** should improve your appearance and sense of wellbeing enormously, but if you insist on fuelling your body with a truck-load of chips and chocolate and your daily workout is walking to the car, you will never achieve more than a fraction of your potential to look your best. Not only that but your energy levels will be much lower than they could be and you will be far more likely to suffer from the negative effects of stress.

What you put in your body and how much you exercise are far more important to the way you appear than the skin cream you use or whether you regularly trim your nasal hair. The good news is that even small changes in your routine – like walking quickly for 20 minutes a day and not drinking alcohol for a couple of days each week – will give enormous improvements to your sense of wellbeing, your general health and how you look.

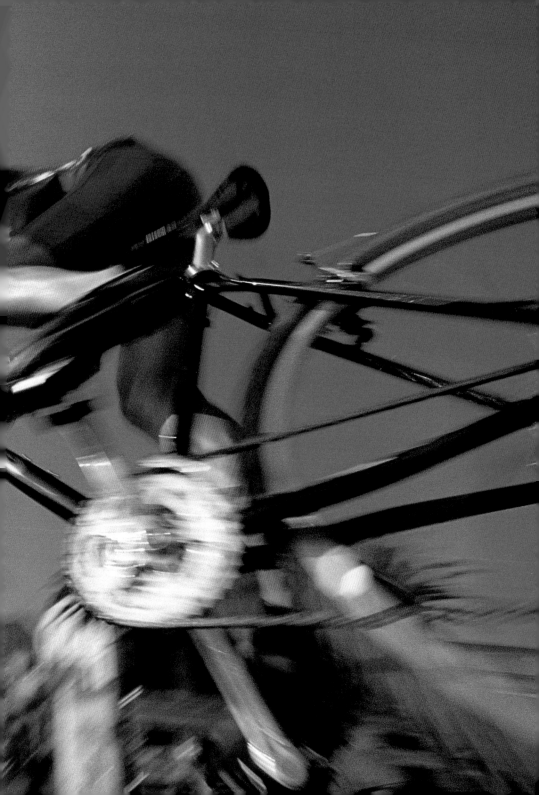

Exercise

Not exercising is like having a Ferrari Testarrossa in your garage, which you tenderly polish and wax but never take on the road – the engine will deteriorate through lack of use. Studies at the Cooper Institute for Aerobic Research in the USA concluded that those who did no exercise were one and a half times more likely to die prematurely than fit people. The benefits of even minimal exercise, such as a brisk 20-minutes walk three times a week, can reduce the risk of heart disease and give you a greater sense of wellbeing, which helps eradicate negative feelings of anxiety and stress. If that is not incentive enough Matt Roberts, a London-based personal trainer, says: 'Exercise promotes a higher level of blood flow around the body and, as fitness levels improve and demand for blood in the body increases, the body adapts by developing new capillaries, which are directly linked to the quality of your skin and hair. Increased levels of oxygen (which is always a key change in someone who exercises) are associated with an improvement in all bodily functions, so anything from hair development to nail growth will be improved.'

Researchers at the University of Wisconsin have discovered that the more oxygen you take in, the less likely you are to suffer from free-radical damage (see page 51), which is linked to premature ageing. Aerobic exercise – brisk walking, jogging or running, bicycling or swimming (why not take up disco dancing?) – will stimulate the circulation, help a sluggish digestion to rid your system of waste and toxins, and bring a healthy glow to your skin. Exercise also helps to stimulate sex and steroid hormones, and is one of the most effective ways of dispelling stress, which can undermine all your good intentions for your skin.

If you are worried about exercise causing you injury, remember that 80 per cent of people visiting physiotherapists do so because of problems caused by immobility rather than due to exercise itself.

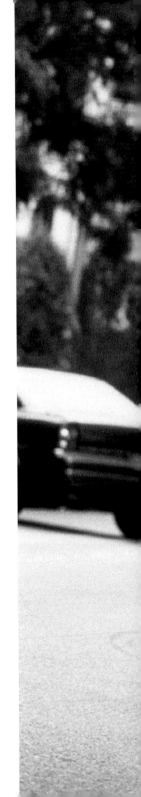

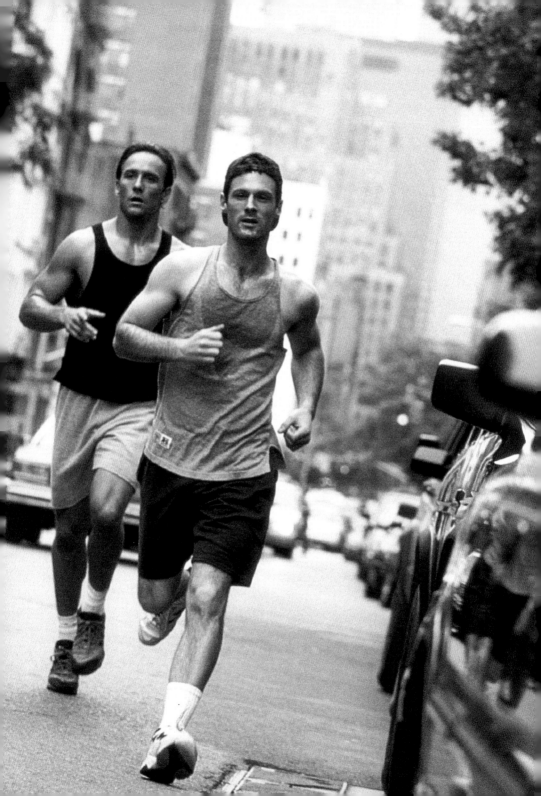

MATT ROBERTS'S HOME WORKOUT ROUTINE

You do not have to spend hours pumping iron in the gym every day or run around your local park ten times each morning before work to get sufficient exercise. It is possible to achieve and maintain a reasonable level of fitness in and around your own home with very little or even no special equipment apart form a good pair of cross-trainers (sports shoes that are suitable for a range of activities). The following workout is composed of three parts – aerobic, resistance and, finally, stretching. Each part is as important as the others to obtain a balanced and complete workout. Ideally, you should try to do some exercise three times a week on non-consecutive days.

AEROBIC work is anything that gets the heart rate and breathing going. Go out into the park to walk, jog or run; dig out your bike or exercise bike; skip or even jog on the spot. Aim to do about 20 minutes of continuous exercise – the first five minutes should be a gentle warm-up to loosen the muscles and the remaining 15 minutes should be at the intensity at which you would just be able to maintain a conversation. As you get fitter, increase the intensity and/or the duration.

RESISTANCE work strengthens your muscles and tones them, improving your overall shape and posture. (Aim to create an inverted V-shape – the most athletic figure – with broad shoulders and a firm waist.) Resistance work will also keep your heart rate raised, continuing a degree of aerobic conditioning. You will need a pair of hand weights (or full beer cans) for these exercises. The number of repetitions is only a guide; if you find any exercise too easy, increase the number of repetitions. Aim to complete the circuit twice. Do not rest between exercises, but take a break of one to two minutes between the circuits. (This routine works well if you are travelling and cannot get to a gym.)

STRETCHING is the unsung hero of all exercise and its importance is becoming increasingly recognized in many sports as a way of avoiding injuries, such as strained ligaments, as well as enabling your body to perform a wider range of movements safely. Ideally you should stretch all the major muscle groups after your warm up before the rest of your workout and then again when you have finished, but if you are pushed for time just stretch after working out as part of your cooling-down routine.

1 PRESS-UPS (20 REPETITIONS) Lie face down on the floor with your toes curled under. With your hands shoulder-width apart and upper arms parallel to the floor, push your body up. Keep your body flat and do not lock your arms when you are furthest from the floor. For a more punishing variation, clap your hands at the top of each push-up.

2 SQUATS (20 REPETITIONS) Stand with your feet facing forward, shoulder-width apart. Bend your knees until your thighs are parallel to the ground, hold, then push up. Face forward at all times.

3 CHAIR DIPS (20 REPETITIONS) Support your body weight with both hands on the edge of a sturdy chair with your heels on the ground and knees slightly bent. Start with straight arms and slowly bend them until your forearms are parallel to the floor, then push up without locking your elbows.

4 LUNGES (20 REPETITIONS) Stand with your feet together, holding weights in both hands. Take a large step forward with one foot and bend your knees until your back knee is almost touching the floor, then step back, keeping your knees slightly bent and your feet pointing forward. Do the same with the other foot.

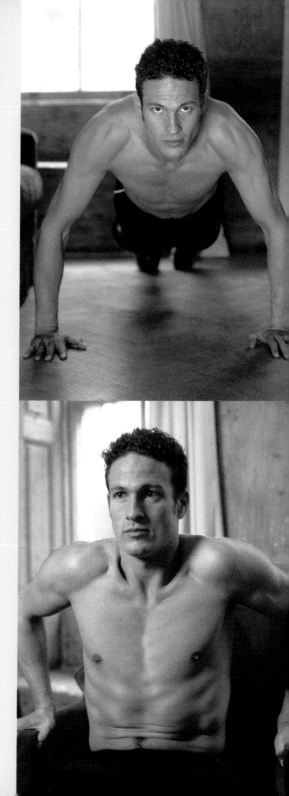

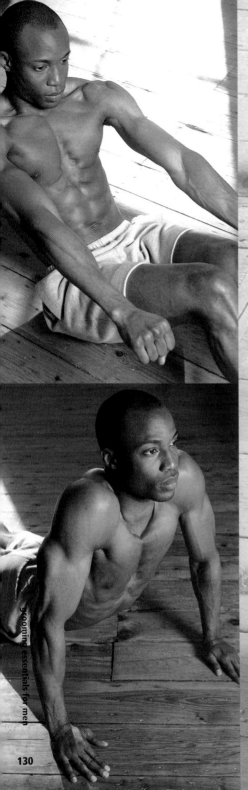

5 OVERHEAD PRESS (20 REPETITIONS) Holding weights in both hands, start with arms bent and hands at shoulder height. Raise your arms together, then return them to the start position.

6 HAMMER CURL (20 REPETITIONS) Standing with your arms by your side and weights in each hand, bend alternate arms towards your shoulder and return them to your side.

7 CRUNCHES (20 REPETITIONS) Lie on your back on a towel with your knees bent and your feet on the floor. Hold your arms out in front of you or, with your elbows pointing outwards, lightly support your head with your fingertips. Raise your head, shoulders and upper back, crunch towards your knees, then lower your body, keeping your head and shoulders off the floor.

8 OBLIQUE CRUNCHES (20 REPETITIONS) In the same position as above, twist towards alternate knees as you crunch to tighten your sides.

9 STRETCH (2 REPETITIONS) Sit on the floor with your legs straight out in front of you with your feet flexed. Raise your arms above your head and slowly lower your torso onto your legs, reaching for your feet with your hands. Hold for three deep breaths. Then lie face down on the floor with your hands under your shoulders. Slowly lift your chest off the floor, keeping your elbows slightly bent. Hold, then slowly lower.

grooming essentials for men

MATT ROBERTS'S TOP SIX EXERCISE TIPS

1 To gain the greatest benefit, exercise at between 75 and 80 per cent of your maximum heart level (the maximum is roughly 220 minus your age. For example, if you are 35 years old, your maximum rate is 185 heart beats per minute, so you should aim for a constant 136 beats per minute during your aerobic exercise (75 per cent of your maximum).

2 Interval training rather than constant pace training is of far greater benefit for heart capacity gains and for fat reduction than consistent pace training, so rather than slogging away non-stop for 30 minutes at the same pace, break up your routine into 15 one-minute high intensity blasts with a one-minute rest in between each blast.

3 Focus on your major muscle groups when doing weight training, which allows you to burn more calories and develop a better body shape. The best muscle groups to focus on are your pectorals, laterals, quadriceps, hamstrings, abdominals and lumbar muscles.

4 Always warm up adequately; not only does it make working out safer, it also improves your ability to exercise when you get down to the real work. Take at least eight minutes to warm up and ideally 12 minutes until your heart is pushed to 85 per cent of its maximum.

5 Never forget to stretch thoroughly after exercise. Remember, half of all back pain is caused by stiff hamstrings. Stretching is also a great way of de-stressing and will help loosen any tense muscles. Breathe steadily through your nose during each movement – it will help you to increase the stretch – and make sure that every breath you take fills the whole of your lungs.

6 Before, during and after your workout take regular breaks to drink water. It is far better to drink small amounts frequently than one large glass, since it will pass through your system quicker.

Water water everywhere

Men drink a total of around 40,000 litres (8,800 gallons) of water in their lifetime. Start missing out on this health essential and some pretty nasty side effects can occur. With two per cent dehydration you will suffer from a 20 per cent reduction in your working capacity, while at ten per cent dehydration more severe symptoms will appear as your thermo-regulation systems break down, leaving you unable to regulate your body's temperature. Double that amount of dehydration and death is imminent. So try to drink a couple of litres of still, room-temperature mineral or filtered water every day to stave off dehydration.

The worrying thing is that according to a recent report many of our work-places are seriously dehydrated, with some having less than 25 per cent hydration (equivalent to the Sahara) and others having humidity levels dryer than Death Valley. This can cause everything from headaches and sore eyes to dry, flaking skin and chapped lips. In such arid conditions, drinking enough water is not just advisable but necessary. So insist that your company installs a water fountain and keep a spring-water face spray handy for when your face feels like it is about to crack.

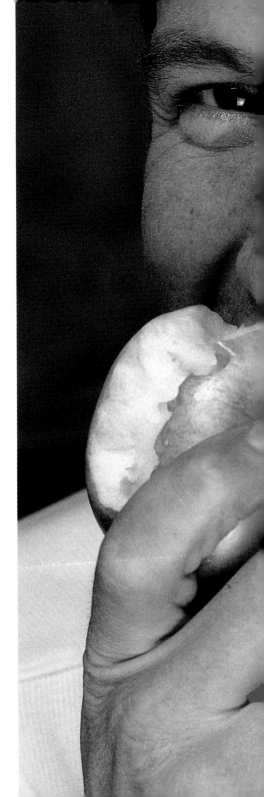

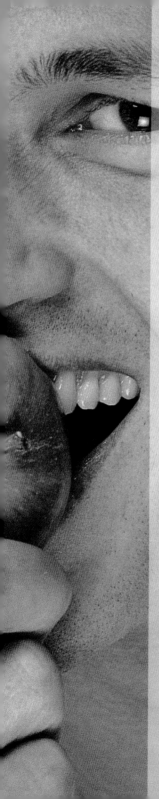

Optimum fuel

Dermatologists are still not agreed to what extent the food you eat affects the general state of your skin, although the connection between specific foods and skin reactions, including rashes, itching and eczema, is certain. A diet rich in fresh foods – particularly fruit, vegetables and grains – and low in processed and refined foods will benefit your whole body, most noticeably your skin.

Healthy skin is dependent on the efficient functioning of the kidneys, intestines and liver. The liver not only manufactures the substances that help remove waste products from the body, but also filters out any harmful chemicals from processed food and drink, alcohol, prescription drugs, and the toxins produced in the body by bacteria and viruses. A sluggish system that allows all these toxins to create havoc in the body can leave your skin looking pasty and blemished.

If you are unsure whether you are getting enough nutrients and vitamins from your diet, supplements can help. The key benefactors to skin are vitamins B6, C, E and zinc (which helps the absorption of vitamin C).

Few of us manage to eat a genuinely balanced diet rich in all the vitamins, minerals and elements needed for optimum health. Our lives are becoming increasingly hectic and stressful; we live in polluted environments and our idea of a varied diet may well be alternating Chinese, Indian and Italian takeaways, without giving vegetables or fruit a look in. If you are concerned about your nutrition, taking daily multivitamin and mineral supplements can only benefit you. Here are a list of the important vitamins and minerals, where to find them in your diet and how much you should be taking on a daily basis.

BETA CAROTENE

There is no bare minimum but Beta Carotene is an effective antioxidant.
FIND IT IN: carrots, sweet potatoes, broccoli, green leafy vegetables, mangoes and apricots.

CHROMIUM

MINIMUM: 25 micrograms
FIND IT IN: meat (especially liver), wholegrains, yeast and wine.

FOLIC ACID

MINIMUM: 200 micrograms
FIND IT IN: dark green vegetables, Marmite and some breakfast cereals that have added folic acid.

IRON

MINIMUM: 9 mg
FIND IT IN: red meat, fish, pulses, dark green vegetables, nuts and seeds.

POTASSIUM

MINIMUM: 3,500 mg
FIND IT IN: bananas, watercress, cabbage, courgettes and mushrooms.

SELENIUM

MINIMUM: 70 micrograms
FIND IT IN: wholegrain cereals and brazil nuts.

VITAMIN B1

MINIMUM: 1 mg
FIND IT IN: lean meat, liver, eggs, wholegrains and milk.

VITAMIN B2

MINIMUM: 1.3 mg
FIND IT IN: wholegrains, yeast, liver, eggs and milk.

VITAMIN B6

MINIMUM: 1.4 mg
FIND IT IN: meat, poultry and eggs.

VITAMIN C

MINIMUM: 40 mg
FIND IT IN: nearly all fruits and their juices, especially citrus fruits, papaya, pears, strawberries, blackcurrants and kiwi fruit.

VITAMIN E

MINIMUM: 4 mg
FIND IT IN: avocado, dark green vegetables, wheatgerm, sunflower seeds, sesame seeds and nuts.

ZINC

MINIMUM: 10 mg
FIND IT IN: breakfast cereal, wholegrain bread, red meat and shellfish, especially oysters.

BALANCED DIETS

Amanda Ursell, a state-registered dietician, recommends the best diets to combat stress, boost your immune system and to supplement an exercise-heavy lifestyle.

DIET TO COUNTERACT STRESS Eat 100 per cent wholemeal bread and wholegrain versions of pasta and rice. These foods are rich in B vitamins, which are needed to keep the nerves in good condition. Avoid too many stimulants, such as coffee, tea and cola drinks. Camomile tea has a calming effect and helps you sleep well, and lettuce also has a mildly sedative effect, so try to include salad in your evening meal.

DIET TO STRENGTHEN YOUR IMMUNE SYSTEM Increase your intake of vitamin C by eating oranges, kiwi fruit, berries of all types, peppers and dark green leafy vegetables like watercress and spinach. Guava and papaya are two particularly rich sources, and fresh citrus-fruit juices also contain immune-boosting vitamin C. Try to eat some red meat, shellfish (especially oysters) and wholegrain cereals; all contain the mineral zinc, which is needed for boosting the immune system.

MUSCLE-BUILDING DIET Make sure that 60–70 per cent of calories in your diet come from carbohydrates. These provide fuel for the muscles, allowing them to exercise and increase in bulk. You also need an adequate supply of lean protein to maintain muscle. So make sure meals and snacks include bread, rice, pasta, potatoes, breakfast cereals and fruit, and that main meals also have some turkey, chicken, fish, dairy produce or pulses.

AMANDA URSELL'S TOP FOUR TIPS FOR HEALTHY EATING

1   Eat a variety of foods, including five 80-g (3-oz) servings of fruit and vegetables daily.

2   Have wholegrain foods instead of refined, white versions whenever possible.

3   Choose lean cuts of meat and reduced-fat dairy products.

4   Only eat fats, oils, lard, margarine and butter and foods containing them in strict moderation and go easy on foods rich in refined sugars.

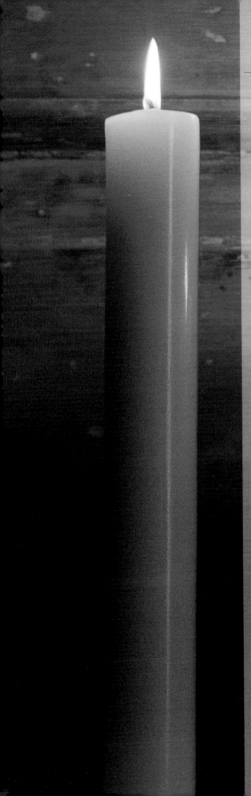

Get rid of stress

Stress is a tricky subject, as some stress is good and necessary while too much of it is most definitely bad. We need stress to get us out of bed in the morning, to push and challenge ourselves in work and play, but too much – and it is a fine line – can lead to a host of negative effects. Sleep may be disrupted, breathing may become shorter and irritability sets in; we may lose our appetites or go on pig-out binges or turn to alcohol or drugs as an escape route. It is important to learn to control levels of stress because, apart from the negative effects on our health, it will seriously undermine all our efforts in the realm of grooming. An ancient proverb states: 'A strung-out individual does not a well-turned-out man make.'

STRETCH AWAY STRESS

Here are six simple stretches, which can be done at your desk or whenever you feel things getting on top of you. Remember to breathe deeply and regularly through your nose throughout the exercises and hold each position for ten deep breaths. Also, focus on what you are doing rather than letting random thoughts enter your head (noticing the difference in temperature in the air as you breathe in and then breathe out can be good at focusing your mind) – and flick off the Pamela Anderson web site.

1   **LOWER BACK STRETCH** Sit up straight in your chair. With both hands, grab your left leg under the knee. Keep your right foot flat on the floor. With your left leg bent, slowly pull that leg toward your chest, hold it for ten breaths, then switch sides. This stretch also loosens your hamstrings.

2   **MID-BACK STRETCH** Interlock your fingers behind your head and gently push your elbows back forcing your shoulder blades together, and hold. Repeat with your fingers interlocking with the other side of the hands uppermost, and hold.

3   **BACK AND SHOULDER STRETCH** To lengthen and release your back, place your hands at shoulder-width apart and at shoulder height flat against a wall and lower your body forward, bending at the hips, until your torso is parallel to the ground; do not let your head drop and hold the position for ten breaths.

4   **NECK STRETCH** This is a great exercise if you have been hunched over your desk and you can feel the tightness across your shoulders and around the base of your neck. Stand or sit straight with your hands behind your back. With your right hand, hold onto your left wrist and gently pull your left arm down and across your back. Tilt your head to the right, lowering your ear to your shoulder. Do not raise your shoulder. Hold for ten breaths, then switch sides and repeat.

5   **HAND STRETCH** If your hands become knotted or tense, stand up and hold your left arm straight in front of you. Put your left hand up and flex the palm away from you, with your right hand gently flex the fingers of your left hand towards you and hold. Switch hands and repeat the stretch.

6   **FACIAL GRIMACE** A yoga exercise called 'The Lion' will relax frown lines and make your face look human again, instead of like a bunched-up fist. Raise your eyebrows as if in surprise and open your eyes wide. Next, open your mouth wide as if to yawn and stick out your tongue as far as possible. Take a deep breath and breathe out quickly through your mouth, relax your face and repeat. Try to avoid doing this exercise in a restaurant or in front of your parents-in-law.

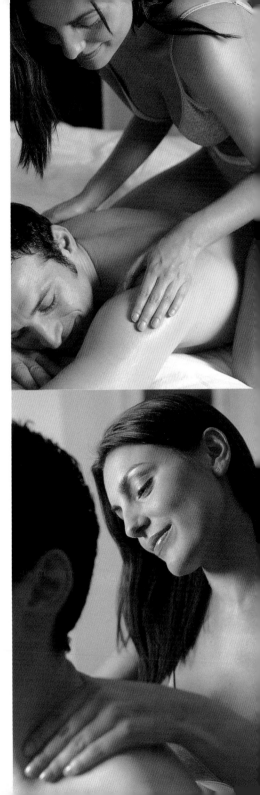

RELAXATION & MASSAGE

Taking time to wind down is one of the most important things you can do to keep yourself in good health. You need to give your brain a proper break from work and any other worries that you may have on a regular basis. This will keep you happier, less agitated and more able to cope with pressure without losing your rag.

One of the best ways to relax is to have an aromatherapy massage, since the soothing physical action eases tired muscles and releases tension, while the essential oils (see page 103) have an uplifting effect on the emotions and help relieve anxiety. Essential oils – the pure, highly concentrated essences that are extracted from the flowers, leaves, stems or roots of plants – have been used for centuries for their therapeutic effects on both the mind and body. For massage, only a few drops of essence are needed, and these should be diluted in a vegetable base oil, such as sweet almond oil, before coming into contact with the skin. During massage, the tiny essential oil molecules are absorbed directly through the skin and the capillaries in the lungs as the vapours are inhaled, and from there they enter the bloodstream. For the greatest benefit, visit a qualified aromatherapist or buy a good step-by-step massage book.

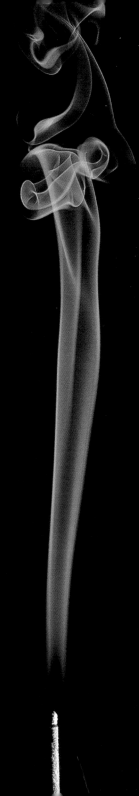

SIX STRESS-BUSTERS

1 **CHILL OUT** When you get home from work have a shower or bath and get changed into comfortable casual clothes to make the break from your work mode.

2 **NO JUNK** If your idea of the perfect evening is junk food, a couple of beers and wall-to-wall television, think again – you are just drugging yourself and increasing toxin levels in your body.

3 **TURN IT OFF** Watch less than five hours of television per week and you will be amazed by how much extra time you have to yourself – time to learn a new skill or read, which is far more relaxing.

4 **QUALITY LEISURE** You need time off in order to be more productive. Go for a walk, read or meditate in order to be more efficient when you are busy.

5 **GET FIT** Exercise is a great way of relieving stress and tension.

6 **TAKE A VACATION** But do not try to pack in too much. It is far better to get up late and immerse yourself in a book or visit a few sights, rather than setting a hectic agenda that will leave you even more exhausted than before you left home.

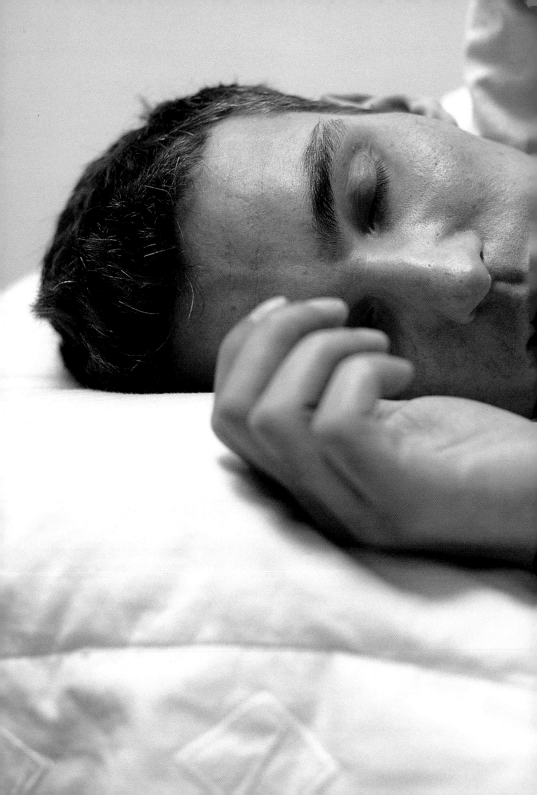

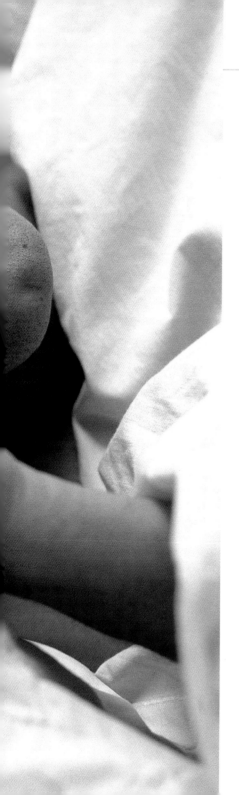

Sleep it off

If you do not get enough sleep you will soon end up looking like one of Dracula's victims. Blood is redirected away from your skin to your exhausted vital organs, leaving your face gaunt with dark circles under your eyes. Lack of sleep adversely affects your memory recall and powers of concentration, too, so you will perform less efficiently at work. Also, some dermatologists assert that during hours of sleep, skin cells replicate faster than at other times and growth hormones are released, which improve both collagen and keratin production.

If you find restful sleep elusive, try going to bed at a regular time to get into a good sleep routine. Avoid caffeine from late afternoon onwards (even tea and chocolate contain caffeine). Camomile tea is a great sleep enhancer, although some people claim it is like drinking a lawn. Alcohol can make sleep erratic and although it may help you fall asleep initially, you will not have as restful a night as you would without it. Regular exercise should help your sleep pattern as it stops the build-up of stress hormones that interfere with easy sleeping. A warm (not hot) bath with a few drops of a relaxing essential oil like sandalwood, lavender or frankincense may help, too.

resources

Acne Support Group
PO Box 230
Hayes
Middlesex
UB4 9HW
Tel 0181 561 6868

Aveda
Tel 0171 410 1600
for stockists

**Barkers and selected
House of Fraser stores**
Tel 0171 937 5432

Bodum
Tel 01451 810460
for stockists

**British Association
of Electrolysis**
For practitioners, send
an SAE to:
2a Tudor Way
Hillingdon, Uxbridge
Middlesex UB10 9AB
Tel 01895 239966

Clarins Gold Salon
Tel 0171 629 2979
for branches

Clinique for Men
Tel 0171 493 9271
for stockists

Commes des Garçons
Tel 01372 275932
for stockists

Cussons
Tel 0161 491 8000
for stockists

Czech & Speake
Tel 0800 919728
for stockists

Decleor Gold Salon
Tel 0171 262 0403
for branches

E'Spa Salon
Tel 01252 741600
for branches

Gap
Tel 0800 427789
for stockists

Gillette
Tel 0181 847 7800
for stockists

Society of Homeopaths
For practitioners, send an SAE to:
2 Artizan Road
Gravesend
Kent DA12 5DZ
Tel 01474 560336

**Ian Matthews
Barbers & Perfumers**
28 Maddox Street
London W1R 9PF
Tel 0171 499 4904

**International Federation
of Aromatherapy**
Stamford House
2-4 Chiswick High Road
London W4 1TH
Tel 0181 742 2605

Molten Brown
Tel 0171 499 6474
Mail-order 0171 625 6550

Muji
Tel 0171 323 2208
for branches

Nicky Clarke For Men
Tel 0171 491 4700
for salon/stockists

Nivea for Men
Tel 0121 327 4750
for stockists

Oral B
Tel 0181 847 7800
for stockists

Philosophy
Space NK   Tel 0171 379 7030
Harrods   Tel 0171 730 1234
Liberty   Tel 0171 734 1234

**Society of Chiropodists
and Podiatrists**
For practitioners, send
an SAE to:
53 Welbeck Street,
London W1M 7HE
Tel 0171 486 3381

Ted Baker
Tel 01372 275932
for stockists

The Body Shop
Customer services
Tel 01903 731500

Tommy Gun
Tel 0171 439 0777
for stockists/mail-order

Wilkinson Sword
Tel 01494 533300

index

acknowledgements

The author would like to thank Alfie, Miss Gina Gibbons and Patsy
for their love and support.

The Publishers would like to thank the shops, salons, health and cosmetic associations and product suppliers (listed on page 142) for lending props and donating grooming products for the shoot. We would also like to thank Jason Bell for providing his Soho flat as a location for photography and C P Hart for the use of their bathroom showroom. Also thanks to Steve Hibbs for lending us a significant part of his wardrobe.

The publishers would like to thank the following sources for their kind
permission to reproduce the pictures in this book:

All Action 7, 73

Famous/AVTA 7, 33t/Hubert Boesl 63/Fred Duval 9bl

Image Bank 108, 110

Jonathan McCree 30

Retna 7, 8t, 8bl, 8br, 9br, 31bl, 31tr, 32br, 33b, 62, 72tr, 72tl

Rex 32bl, 74bl, 75t, 75br

Vin Mag Archive 6

Every effort has been made to acknowledge correctly and contact the source and/copyright holder of each picture, and Carlton Books Limited apologizes for any unintentional errors or omissions which will be corrected in future editions of this book.

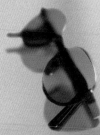